Hon...   ...cology

Ulster Hospital, Dundonald, Northern Ireland

ARNOLD

A member of the Hodder Headline Group
LONDON

First published in Great Britain in 2003 by
Arnold, a member of the Hodder Headline Group,
338 Euston Road, London NW1 3BH

http://www.arnoldpublishers.com

Distributed in the United States of America by
Oxford University Press Inc.,
198 Madison Avenue, New York, NY10016
Oxford is a registered trademark of Oxford University Press

Whilst the advice and information in this book are believed to be true and
accurate at the date of going to press, neither the authors nor the publisher
can accept any legal responsibility or liability for any errors or omissions
that may be made. In particular (but without limiting the generality of the
preceding disclaimer) every effort has been made to check drug dosages;
however, it is still possible that errors have been missed. Furthermore,
dosage schedules are constantly being revised and new side effects
recognized. For these reasons the reader is strongly urged to consult the
drug companies' printed instructions before administering any of the drugs
recommended in this book.

British Library Cataloguing in Publication Data
A catalogue record for this book is available from the British Library

Library of Congress Cataloging-in-Publication Data
A catalog record for this book is available from the Library of Congress

ISBN 0 340 80926 4

1 2 3 4 5 6 7 8 9 10

Commissioning Editor: Joanna Koster
Production Editor: Wendy Rooke
Production Controller: Bryan Eccleshall
Cover Design: Mousemat

Typeset in 10/12 Minion by Phoenix Photosetting, Chatham, Kent
Printed and bound in Malta

What do you think about this book? Or any other Arnold title? Please send your comments to
feedback.arnold@hodder.co.uk

Contents

Preface

The MRCOG Part 2 exam is constantly changing, and it is now very structured and systematic. Although a wide understanding of both the theory and practice is essential, candidates must also practise the technique of the exam, which is equally important.

The 800 MCQs in this book have been designed to test your theoretical and practical knowledge of obstetrics and gynaecology as recommended in the syllabus for the exam. The layout is similar to the layout currently used in the part 2 exam. The answers are detailed and are drawn from current literature (*British Journal of Gynaecology, British Medical Journal, The Obstetrician and Gynaecologist*, RCOG Guidelines), Cochrane database and the Progress series. Some of the answers are 'augmented' with additional, relevant information (see boxed text in Answers section).

The CD-ROM that you received with the book is a novel aid to learning, and will help you to practise the essential technique. The questions can be selected at random to create a practice paper which you can sit under 'examination conditions'. After the mock examination the program will calculate your score. The questions will appear in a different order every time. The answers and augmentations are the same as appear in the text. Alternatively, you may use the CD-ROM to answer questions one at a time or in small blocks and refer to the answers as you go along. If you wish, you can also keep a running total score.

Whether you prefer the text or the CD-ROM they will help you to prepare for the part 2 examination and, I hope, pass.

Good luck!

R de C-W,
B McE,
K El-H,
TA and BA
for the OGWW Team.

Acknowledgements

We would like to acknowledge the invaluable assistance of
Joanne McAleese – computer programmer and secretary to OGWW.

Questions

1. The risk of familial ovarian cancer is high if:

A. Two first-degree relatives have ovarian cancer.
B. One woman has ovarian cancer and a first-degree relative under 50 years of age has breast cancer.
C. The BRCA1 gene is detected.
D. One woman has ovarian cancer and two first-degree relatives have breast cancer diagnosed before 60 years of age.
E. One woman has ovarian cancer and three first-degree relatives have colorectal cancer with at least one case diagnosed before 50 years of age.

2. The following substances are safe in pregnancy:

A. Chlorpheniramine.
B. Aspirin.
C. Vitamin A.
D. Vitamin D.
E. Polio vaccination.
F. Tuberculosis vaccination.

3. Malpresentations:

A. Face presentation is a contraindication to vacuum extraction.
B. Asynclitism occurs when the vertex fails to descend with the sagittal suture in the transverse diameter of the pelvis.
C. Persistent occipitoposterior (OP) position may occur if the vertex remains deflexed on entering the pelvis.
D. Persistent anterior cervical lip is a sign of persistent OP position.

4. Uterovaginal prolapse:

A. Nagel exercises aim to contract the pubococcygeus in order to improve the symptoms attributable to a cystocele.
B. First-degree prolapse describes protrusion of the cervix through the vaginal introitus.
C. Colpocliesis is commonly used to repair a rectocele.
D. Rectocele presents as a protrusion of the anterior vaginal wall.
E. Prolapse cannot occur after hysterectomy.
F. The pelvic floor muscles form a gutter sloping downwards and forwards.
G. Procidentia describes descent of the anterior vaginal wall through the vaginal introitus.
H. Urethrocele describes prolapse of the lowest third of the anterior vaginal wall.
I. Prolapse of the pouch of Douglas is called an enterocele.
J. Vaginal hysterectomy is the treatment of choice for procidentia in a patient fit for theatre.
K. Rectocele is the commonest form of prolapse.
L. Ring pessaries rest within the posterior fornix and over the symphysis pubis.
M. A Manchester repair involves cervical amputation and anterior and posterior repairs.
N. An enterocele contains small bowel or omentum.

5. The following drugs are known teratogens:

A. Danazol.
B. Warfarin.
C. Methotrexate.
D. Tetracycline.
E. Lithium.

6. In the treatment of eclampsia:

A. Phenytoin is the anticonvulsant of choice.
B. Magnesium sulphate is less efficient than phenytoin at preventing recurrent seizures.
C. Diazepam has no place in modern management.
D. Hydralazine is used in preference to labetalol to control severe hypertension.
E. The use of labetalol may cause fetal distress.

7. Hair:

A. The cyclical phases of growth take up to 6 months.
B. Hair grows at a rate of 1 mm per month.
C. Androgens provoke terminal hair growth on the scalp.
D. Lanugo hair may be seen in women with anorexia nervosa.
E. Acanthosis nigricans is normally found on the face and trunk.
F. Hypertrichosis is excessive growth of fine vellus hair.
G. Hypertrichosis responds well to anti-androgens.

8. Neonatal lupus erythematosus (NLE):

A. Is probably due to fetal antibodies.
B. Incidence: 1:2000 live births.
C. Characterized by scaling annular or elliptical plaques on the extremities.

9. Diagnosis of preterm labour:

A. The presence of fibronectin in cervical samples means that the onset of labour is less likely.
B. Home uterine activity monitoring has been proven to decrease preterm deliveries.
C. In cases of spontaneous rupture of the membranes at term, diagnosis by nitrazene swabs is accurate in more than 95 per cent of cases.

10. Group B haemolytic *Streptococcus* (GBS)

A. Is a facultative aerobic organism.
B. Is an encapsulated bacillus.
C. Stains Gram positive.
D. Is usually arranged in chains on Gram stain.
E. Definitive identification is based on microscopic examination of material suspended in 10 per cent potassium hydroxide.
F. The gastro-intestinal tract is the major primary reservoir.

11. Recognized risk factors for placental abruption include:
A. Increasing parity.
B. Cocaine use.
C. Preterm premature rupture of membranes.
D. Cigarette smoking.
E. Maternal anxiety.
F. Fibroids underneath the placenta.
G. Advanced age.

12. Fetal well-being:
A. In the second half of pregnancy fetal growth is determined to a greater degree by environmental factors than by genetic factors.
B. Male babies weigh more than female babies on average at term.
C. Smoking marijuana during pregnancy is associated with maternal hypotension.
D. Smoking marijuana during pregnancy is associated with a low birth weight (LBW) baby.
E. Regarding Doppler studies of the placenta, a dichotic notch in the uterine artery waveform is indicative of low resistance within the vessel.
F. Birth weight tends to decrease from the first to the second pregnancies.

13. Dichorionic twin pregnancy:
A. The incidence of fetal abnormality is no different per fetus compared to a singleton pregnancy.
B. Different-sex fetuses are always dichorionic.
C. The rate of fetal loss before 24 weeks is 12 per cent.

14. Vacuum extraction:
A. The incidence of neonatal scalp injuries is not related to the type of vacuum extractor cup.
B. The recommended operating vacuum pressure is between 6.0 and 8.0 kgm/cm^2.
C. The flexion point is located 2 cm anterior to the posterior fontanelle.
D. The desired vacuum pressure may be achieved in one step and traction commenced after 2 min.

15. Endometriosis:
A. 65 per cent of patients have ovarian involvement.
B. Biopsies of suspicious tissue must include endometrial stroma and glands in order to diagnose the condition.
C. Disease severity is an indicator of the amount of pain experienced by the patient.
D. The incidence is highest in those investigated for chronic abdominal pain.
E. Commonly presents with superficial dyspareunia.
F. Findings are constant throughout the affected population.
G. Is easily diagnosed by clinical examination in an outpatient setting.
H. Fixed retroversion of the uterus is a variant of normal.

16. Thalidomide:
A. Is a hypnotic/sedative drug.
B. Maternal ingestion has resulted in the teratogenic effect known as phocomelia.
C. Phocomelia is absence of the short bones of the upper and/or lower limbs.
D. Is used in the treatment of tuberculosis.

17. In the infant of the diabetic mother:
A. The incidence of respiratory distress syndrome is increased because insulin antagonizes the action of cortisol on sphingomyelin synthesis.
B. The presence of acidic phospholipid phosphatidylglycerol (PG) is a final marker of fetal lung maturity.
C. Respiratory distress syndrome may occur despite a 'mature' lecithin:sphingomyelin ratio (>2).

18. Placenta accreta:
A. The optimum management is Caesarean hysterectomy.
B. Is commonly associated with placenta praevia.
C. Is associated with placenta praevia in over 50 per cent of cases.

19. Diabetes mellitus in pregnancy:
A. Is defined if the 2-h glucose is >11 mmol/L.
B. During labour, glucose should be given as a vehicle for an oxytocin infusion.
C. During labour, blood glucose concentration should be maintained <7 mmol/L.
D. In pregnancy, there is an increased glucose concentration in the vaginal epithelium.
E. Pre-eclampsia is seen in 8 per cent of pregnant patients with diabetes mellitus.
F. The rate of congenital malformations is increased by a factor of 10.

20. Endometrial carcinomas in association with oestrogen therapy:
A. Are well differentiated.
B. Are deeply invasive.
C. Are sensitive to progestogen therapy.
D. Generally have a poor prognosis.
E. Have a high recurrence rate.

21. Hypertension:
A. Hypertension is an uncommon complication of pregnancy.
B. The diastolic blood pressure (DBP) in pregnancy corresponds to the appearance of the Korotkoff sounds.
C. Only one category of hypertension in pregnancy exists.
D. Transient hypertension is difficult to diagnose clinically.
E. Pregnancy-induced hypertension and transient hypertension are synonymous.
F. Women suffering from chronic hypertension are at no more risk of fetal complications in pregnancy than normotensive patients.
G. Fetal complications in patients with chronic hypertension are preventable.

22. Ovarian cancer: the following statements are true:

A. Separate International Federation of Obstetrics and Gynaecology (FIGO) staging systems exist for epithelial and sex-cord/stromal ovarian tumours.

B. Granulosa cell tumours have a high frequency of rupture.

C. Meigs' syndrome consists of ascites, hydrothorax and a malignant ovarian tumour.

D. Metastatic tumours of the ovary commonly originate in the gastro-intestinal tract.

E. Krukenberg tumours are metastatic ovarian neoplasms originating exclusively in the stomach.

23. Progesterone-only contraception:

A. The progesterone-only pill acts by inhibiting ovulation.

B. Depo-Provera (medroxyprogesterone acetate) can suppress pituitary gonadotrophins.

C. Progesterone-only methods that inhibit ovulation increase the risk of functional ovarian cysts.

24. Antibiotics with potential adverse effects on the human fetus include:

A. Chloramphenicol.

B. Co-trimoxazole.

C. Chloroquine.

D. Ticarcillin.

E. Nitrofurantoin.

F. Erythromycin.

G. Fluoroquinolones.

25. On transvaginal ultrasonography:

A. The ventricular system within the head is visible at 8 weeks.

B. The head is not distinguishable from the body until 12 weeks.

C. Physiological herniation of the umbilicus is seen at 9 weeks.

D. In early pregnancy, the ovaries will be seen to contain small primordial follicles.

E. In pregnancy, free fluid in the pouch of Douglas is not a normal finding.

26. Breech presentation is more frequent in the following situations:

A. A septate uterus.

B. Fetal neuromuscular disorders.

C. Hydrocephaly.

D. Anencephaly.

27. Echogenic foci in the fetal heart ('golf ball'):

A. Are found in less than 1 per cent of trisomy 21 (Down's syndrome) fetuses.

B. Have an overall incidence of about 3 per cent.

28. Anaemia in pregnancy:

A. Cardiac output falls in the presence of anaemia.
B. Red blood cells in the pregnant patient have the same haemoglobin concentration as in the non-pregnant patient.
C. Anaemia is diagnosed when the haemoglobin is less than 11 g/dL.
D. Severe anaemia renders the patient more susceptible to puerperal infection.
E. The fetus and placenta require approximately 500 mg of iron per pregnancy.
F. The recommended therapeutic intake of elemental iron is 10 mg per day.
G. Ferric salts are better absorbed than ferrous salts.
H. Iron absorption occurs predominantly in the jejunum.

29. Malignant trophoblastic disease:

A. The risk of choriocarcinoma after a hydatidiform mole is about 2–4 per cent.
B. The sonographic appearance of invasive mole is focal areas of increased echogenicity within the myometrium.
C. The sonographic appearance of placental site trophoblastic tumours is of large, diffuse, fluid-filled cysts.
D. A sonographic picture of a semi-solid echogenic mass is in keeping with choriocarcinoma.

30. Concerning drug use and adverse effects to the fetus:

A. A drug given after 12 weeks' gestation will not produce a major anatomical defect.
B. Prilocaine, if used as a local anaesthetic in epidural infusions, may cause methaemoglobinaemia.
C. Prostaglandin inhibitors may lead to premature closure of the ductus arteriosus.
D. Podophyllum for the treatment of genital warts may cause teratogenesis and fetal death.
E. Cimetidine may have an anti-androgenic effect.
F. Tricyclic antidepressants can cause neonatal tachycardia.

31. Regarding external cephalic version (ECV):

A. The success rate is greatest in the second trimester.
B. The success rate after 37 weeks' gestation is 90 per cent.
C. It carries a significant risk of fetal mortality.
D. Fetal morbidity is usually associated with placental abruption and cord entanglement.

32. Genuine stress incontinence (GSI):

A. More than 150 operations have been described for the treatment of stress incontinence.
B. Anterior colporrhaphy is the operation of choice.
C. After anterior colporrhaphy, de-novo detrusor instability may arise in 50 per cent of cases.
D. Anterior colporrhaphy has success rates of 40–70 per cent.
E. Complications of Marshall–Marchetti Krantz procedure include osteitis pubis in 5 per cent of patients.
F. The Marshall–Marchetti Krantz procedure is a useful operation to correct a cystocele in association with stress incontinence.

33. Folic acid:
A. The folate requirement in pregnancy rises to 350–400 micrograms per day.
B. Megaloblastic anaemia in pregnancy is a common complication.
C. Folic acid utilization is decreased in pregnant patients taking anti-epileptic medication.
D. Megaloblastic anaemia in pregnancy may result in alopecia.
E. Folate levels are not affected by sickle-cell disease.
F. In maternal folate deficiency, the fetus also usually develops folate deficiency.
G. Folate deficiency leads to hyposegmentation of the neutrophils.

34. Urodynamic investigation:
A. The urethral pressure profile is an essential part of urodynamic investigation.
B. If the maximum urethral closing pressure is low (<20 cm H_2O) it may be an indication for a sling procedure.
C. Dipstick testing for nitrites and leukocytes is adequate to exclude urinary tract infection (UTI) prior to commencing the test.
D. The infection rate after urodynamics may be 10 per cent.
E. Genuine stress incontinence (GSI) is diagnosed when urine loss is demonstrated during provocation in the presence of a rise in detrusor pressure.

35. Recurrent miscarriage:
A. Is defined as the loss of three or more pregnancies.
B. Has an incidence of 0.3 per cent.
C. Diabetes mellitus has been associated with recurrent miscarriage.
D. Activated protein C resistance (APCR) is found in 20 per cent of women with a history of recurrent miscarriage.
E. If investigations for recurrent miscarriage are negative, the chance of a live birth in a subsequent pregnancy is 65–70 per cent.
F. An identifiable cause can be found in about 50 per cent of cases.

36. Gastro-intestinal disease and pregnancy:
A. Peptic ulceration is more common during pregnancy.
B. Undiagnosed coeliac disease in pregnant women carries a risk of neural tube defect in the fetus.
C. Exacerbation of inflammatory bowel disease is more likely in pregnancy.

37. Pre-eclampsia:
A. Consists of a triad of elevated blood pressure, proteinuria and oedema in the first trimester.
B. The diagnosis depends on the presence of proteinuria of more than 20 g in more than 24 h.
C. Is less common in black races than in Caucasian.
D. There is no increase in the risk of hypertension in later life.
E. Fibronectin is raised in the first and second trimesters.
F. Elevated plasma uric acid occurs after the development of proteinuria.

38. Detrusor instability:
A. Clam iliocystoplasty is indicated only in idiopathic urgency.
B. Anticholinergic agents are effective but are limited by side effects.
C. Most cases of urinary incontinence are attributed to detrusor instability.
D. Patients often have reduced bladder capacity.
E. Up to 6 per cent of patients have a combination of detrusor instability and urethral sphincter incompetence.

39. The combined oral contraceptive pill aggravates the following conditions:
A. Dysmenorrhoea.
B. Premenstrual tension.
C. Endometriosis.

40. Drug treatment for menorrhagia:
A. Danazol is not associated with any serious side effects.
B. The side effects of danazol are not dose-related.
C. Gonadotrophin-releasing hormone (GnRH) analogues are the medical treatment of choice for menorrhagia.
D. Combined hormone replacement therapy can be given in conjunction with GnRH analogues.
E. GnRH analogues are useful agents in the long-term treatment of menorrhagia.

41. Management of hydatidiform moles:
A. Following a complete mole, approximately 15 per cent of patients need treatment for persistent trophoblastic disease.
B. The combined oral contraceptive pill (COCP) is contraindicated during follow-up in the presence of abnormal human chorionic gonadotrophin (hCG) level (>5 IU/mL).
C. The combined oral contraceptive pill is contraindicated during follow-up in the presence of normal hCG levels.
D. Patients in the low-risk category on the prognostic scoring system for gestational trophoblastic disease are best treated with methotrexate and folinic acid.
E. Myelosuppression is an uncommon side effect of methotrexate.

42. Chemotherapy for breast cancer:
A. Will render all patients infertile.
B. The chance of permanent amenorrhoea is directly related to age.

43. Thrombocytopenia:
A. Thrombocytopenia in pregnancy is always of the autoimmune variety.
B. Autoimmune thrombocytopenia is associated with antiphospholipid antibodies.
C. Autoimmune thrombocytopenia usually deteriorates in pregnancy.
D. Antiplatelet antibodies do not cross the placenta.

44. Diaphragmatic hernia:
A. The defect is usually located on the right side of the diaphragm.
B. Most fetuses are stillborn.

45. Absolute contraindications to the combined oral contraceptive pill (COCP) include:
A. Carcinoma in situ of the cervix.
B. Diabetes mellitus.
C. Anticoagulant medicine.
D. Hypertension.

46. Cardiovascular drugs with possible adverse fetal effects:
A. Amiodarone hydrochloride (anti-arrhythmic) may cause neonatal goitre if given to a mother during pregnancy.
B. Angiotensin-converting enzyme (ACE) inhibitors may affect fetal renal function.
C. Intra-uterine growth retardation may result from using a beta-blocker during pregnancy.
D. Methyldopa may cause a positive Coombs' test in the neonate.

47. Regarding breech presentation:
A. The incidence at term is 40 per cent.
B. At 26–32 weeks approximately 40–50 per cent of all presentations are breech.
C. Only 2 per cent of breech presentations at 29 weeks will convert spontaneously to cephalic presentation by term.
D. Fetuses in the flexed (complete) presentation are more likely to spontaneously convert to cephalic than extended (frank).
E. Occipital diastasis is cerebral damage with spastic cerebral palsy.
F. The incidence of congenital abnormalities is higher than in cephalic presentations.

48. Late-onset neonatal infection with Group B haemolytic *Streptococcus*:
A. Usually presents after more than 7 days, but rarely after the third month.
B. The mortality rate for term infants is 2–8 per cent.
C. The rate of nosocomial transmission is similar to vertical.
D. Over 90 per cent are caused by antigenic subtype III.
E. Over 80 per cent manifest as meningitis.
F. Otitis media may be a finding.
G. The overall mortality rate is 2 per cent.
H. Approximately 50 per cent of survivors have neurological sequelae.

49. Asthma:
A. In the pregnant woman with severe asthma steroids should not be given.
B. Pulmonary embolism can present with bronchospasm.
C. A pregnant patient with asthma has the same chance of having a child who will develop asthma as a non-asthmatic pregnant woman.
D. Induction of labour with dinoprostone is contraindicated because prostaglandin E_2 has a vasoconstrictive effect on the bronchus.

50. Postpartum haemorrhage (PPH):
A. Secondary PPH is classified as occurring between 24 h and 6 months post delivery.
B. Occurs most frequently in the second week of the puerperium.
C. Is a minor cause of maternal mortality.
D. Routine use of oxytocics in the third stage of labour reduces the risk of haemorrhage by 30–40 per cent.

51. Endometriosis and gonadotrophin-releasing hormone (GnRH) agonist treatment:
A. Is associated with reduction in bone mineral density in the first 6 months of treatment.
B. Bone loss is restored within 2 years of treatment cessation.
C. Addback oestrogen therapy reduces the effect of GnRH agonists.
D. Postoperative treatment prolongs the pain free interval after conservative surgery.

52. The following statements are true:
A. The double-bubble appearance on a fetal ultrasound scan indicates duodenal atresia.
B. Trisomy 21 is commonly associated with duodenal atresia.
C. The absence of the stomach bubble in the presence of polyhydramnios is diagnostic of oesophageal atresia.

53. Hyperprolactinaemia:
A. Is a frequent cause of oestrogen-deficient amenorrhoea and infertility.
B. Is associated with hypothyroidism.
C. May be caused by dopamine agonists.
D. Is detrimental to the fetus.
E. Hyperprolactinaemic amenorrhoea may result in reduction in vertebral bone density of almost 25 per cent.

54. HIV-1 infection in pregnancy:
A. The overall risk of transmission for breast-feeding mothers is 10–20 per cent.
B. Serological diagnosis of infection in infants born to HIV-infected mothers is reliable after the first 6 months.
C. Approximately one-half of vertically infected children develop AIDS in the first year of life.
D. Neonatal anaemia is a side effect of zidovudine therapy.
E. All HIV-infected women should be delivered by Caesarean section.
F. HIV-infected women should be advised not to breast-feed if safe alternatives are available.

55. Contraindications to the intra-uterine contraceptive device (IUCD) include:
A. A history of ectopic pregnancy.
B. A history of rheumatic heart disease.
C. A history of valvular heart disease.

56. Early-onset neonatal infection with Group B haemolytic *Streptococcus*:
A. The mean age is day 5 of life.
B. 70–80 per cent occurs in low birth weight (LBW) neonates (<2500 g) and among women with obstetric complications.
C. The majority of neonates present with meningitis.

57. Birth asphyxia that is severe enough to cause hypoxic ischaemic encephalopathy will have:
A. Severe umbilical artery metabolic acidaemia (pH <7.0).
B. A low Apgar score <3 for more than 5 min.
C. Abnormal neurological signs during the neonatal period.
D. Evidence of hypoxic damage to other body systems (cardiovascular, pulmonary, gastrointestinal, renal or haematological).

58. Autoimmune disease:
A. The antibodies involved in maternal myasthenia gravis do not cross the placenta.
B. Rheumatoid arthritis tends to improve during pregnancy.

59. The following are recognized drug side effects:
A. Postmenopausal bleeding with misoprostol.
B. Pyrexia with gemeprost.
C. Hyponatraemia with syntocinon infusion.
D. Tinnitus with ergometrine maleate.
E. Bronchospasm with carboprost.

60. Blood pressure in pregnant patients:
A. Korotkoff V corresponds more closely to intra-arterial pressure.
B. The diastolic pressure in the second trimester is 15 mmHg lower than before pregnancy.
C. Is considered elevated if the systolic reading is more than 140 mmHg or the diastolic reading is more than 90 mmHg.
D. Raised blood pressure complicates between 20 and 25 per cent of pregnancies.
E. Hypertension alone developing after 37 weeks' gestation is not usually associated with an adverse outcome.

61. Multiple pregnancy:
A. The UK incidence of twins is 20 per 1000 pregnancies.
B. 3:1000 of these are monozygous.
C. The incidence of conjoined twins is <1 per cent of overall twins.
D. The timing of separation is usually >14 days.
E. Structural defects in twins are usually concordant.
F. Chorionic villus sampling (CVS) is more appropriate in perinatal diagnosis.
G. Up to 20 per cent of twins diagnosed in the first trimester will proceed only as singletons.
H. In higher multiples fetal reduction may not improve the chance of survival.

62. Thromboembolism in gynaecology:
A. Venous thromboembolism accounts for one-fifth of perioperative hysterectomy deaths.
B. The use of prophylactic heparin in gynaecological surgery is associated with an increase in the incidence of wound haematoma.
C. Use of the combined oral contraceptive pill (COCP) is associated with a higher incidence of perioperative deep venous thromboses (DVP).
D. There is no evidence of an association of hormone replacement therapy (HRT) with venous thromboembolism and HRT need not be stopped prior to surgery.

63. Anatomy and physiology of the female lower urinary tract:
A. In the adult the urinary bladder has a mean volume of 500 mL.
B. The detrusor muscle is innervated by sympathetic nerves S2–S4 and receives a rich efferents supply.
C. Vascular congestion of the submucosal venous plexus contributes to the maintenance of urinary continence.
D. The normal maximum flow rate on urodynamic testing is 5 mL/s.
E. Bladder contractions are caused by stimulation of the sympathetic nervous system.

64. Raloxifene:
A. Is a selective oestrogen receptor modulator.
B. May produce a 42 per cent decrease in the incidence of vertebral fracture.
C. May produce a 76 per cent decrease in new breast cancer.
D. Does not affect the risk of deep venous thrombosis.
E. Helps vasomotor symptoms of the menopause.

65. Systemic lupus erythematosus (SLE):
A. Pregnancy may exacerbate the symptoms of SLE.
B. Is associated with preterm delivery.
C. Vaginal delivery is contraindicated.
D. Neonatal lupus erythematosus is characterized by tachycardia.
E. Heart block in the fetus of a mother with SLE may cause intra-uterine death.

66. Investigations for infertility:
A. When performing a hysterosalpingogram (HSG), water-soluble contrast can give more information than oil-based contrast media.
B. Acute pelvic infection is an absolute contraindication to HSG.
C. The post-coital test is best performed 12 h after intercourse.
D. Normal post-coital test demonstrates more than five motile sperm present per high-power field.

67. Early pregnancy ultrasound:
A. Abdominal grey-scale ultrasound imaging can only detect a gestational sac when the human chorionic gonadotrophin (hCG) level is >6500 IU/L.
B. During fetal development an intra-uterine sac is the first structure to be visualized by transvaginal ultrasound. Next is the fetal echo.
C. Heart motion by transvaginal ultrasound, should always be present by 46 days.
D. At 9 weeks' gestation, the fetal heart beat is 175 beats per minute (bpm).

68. Use of thiazides during pregnancy has been associated with:
A. Permanent neonatal hypoglycaemia.
B. Neonatal thrombocytopenia.
C. Lower maternal blood volume.
D. Body hair abnormalities.
E. Neonatal hyperbilirubinaemia.

69. Primary varicella zoster infection:
A. Pneumonia occurs in 1 per cent of pregnant women with primary varicella zoster infection.
B. Congenital varicella syndrome is secondary to primary varicella zoster infection occurring before 20 weeks' gestation.
C. If the primary maternal infection occurs before 20 weeks' gestation, the risk of congenital varicella syndrome is 20 per cent.

70. Patients with a history of polycystic ovarian disease are at increased risk of:
A. Osteoporosis.
B. Endometrial neoplasia.
C. Late-onset adrenal enzyme deficiencies.
D. Hypertension in pregnant patients.
E. Insulin-dependent diabetes mellitus.

71. Repair of perineal trauma:
A. Vicryl Rapide is fully absorbed within 40 days.
B. There is no difference in the incidence of short-term pain with continuous sutures compared with that using interrupted sutures.
C. Silk sutures are associated with a decreased incidence of perineal pain compared to polyglycolic acid sutures.

72. In cases of recurrence of endometrial carcinoma:
A. 5–10 per cent of treated patients will die within 5 years of diagnosis.
B. The largest percentage of recurrences will be local.
C. The majority of recurrences occur within 1 year.
D. 10 per cent of patients present with recurrence more than 5 years from diagnosis.

73. Hirsutism:
A. Obese people are more prone to hirsutism despite the presence of a normal or serum testosterone.
B. The maximum score on the Ferriman–Galwey scoring system is 44.
C. Prevalence varies according to race.
D. Less than 10 per cent of women with idiopathic hirsutism have polycystic ovarian disease.

74. Regarding the aetiology of human infertility the following are true:
A. Ovulatory dysfunction is the major cause of infertility.
B. Smoking may decrease fertility.
C. Treatment of mild endometriosis enhances infertility.
D. A history of intermenstrual bleeding may suggest the possibility of tubal disease as a cause of infertility.
E. Male factor is responsible for the failure to conceive in fewer than 5 per cent of cases.
F. Hydrosalpinx greater than 3 cm is associated with lower rates of pregnancy even after tubal surgery.

75. Aetiology of preterm labour:
A. A history of premature delivery is a strong risk factor for another premature delivery.
B. Fetal oesophageal atresia has a recognized association with spontaneous preterm labour.
C. Preterm rupture of membranes is responsible for 50 per cent of preterm deliveries.
D. A previous history of preterm labour is a useful predictor in a subsequent pregnancy.
E. Approximately 6–8 per cent of births deliver before 37 weeks.
F. In almost half of the cases of preterm delivery, an underlying cause can be found.
G. Bacteria have been implicated in the pathogenesis of preterm labour because they release prostaglandins directly, which stimulate uterine activity.
H. Bacterial vaginosis in the second trimester is associated with a 2.5-fold increase in preterm birth.

76. Steroids and hormones in pregnancy:
A. The incidence of fetal loss is increased in mothers taking corticosteroids during pregnancy.
B. 12-Hydroxyprogesterone may cause clitoral enlargement in the female fetus.
C. Oestrogens may cause urogenital defects in the male fetus.
D. 19 Nor-steroids are androgenic.

77. The following combinations of disease and inheritance are true:
A. Retinitis pigmentosa: X-linked recessive.
B. Cystic fibrosis: autosomal dominant.
C. Tuberous sclerosis: autosomal recessive.
D. Malignant hyperthermia: autosomal dominant.
E. Phenylketonuria: autosomal dominant.
F. Congenital adrenal hyperplasia: autosomal dominant.
G. Fragile X syndrome: X-linked disorder.
H. Marfan's syndrome: autosomal dominant.
I. Duchenne's muscular dystrophy: X-linked recessive.
J. Von Willebrand's disease: autosomal dominant.
K. Inheritance of thalassaemia is autosomal dominant.

78. Problems at delivery:
A. A nuchal cord describes a cord wrapped around the neck of the fetus.
B. Haemorrhoids complicating vaginal delivery are more common in primiparous patients.
C. Hypertensive disorders of pregnancy causing maternal death are more common in the antenatal period.

79. Treatment of varicella zoster:
A. Acyclovir may be given to pregnant women seen less than 24 h after the development of the varicella rash at any stage of pregnancy.
B. Neonatal infection should be treated with acyclovir.
C. Varicella pneumonia is an indication for oral acyclovir.

80. An increased risk of congenital anomalies is associated with a variety of anticonvulsants:
A.   Carbamazepine may cause neonatal hypothyroidism.
B.   Phenytoin leads to an increased incidence of neural tube defects.
C.   Phenobarbitone is associated with neonatal haemorrhage.
D.   Sodium valproate does not increase the risk of neural tube defects.

81. Regarding the management of thromboembolic disease:
A.   A ventilation–perfusion (VQ) scan for the diagnosis of pulmonary embolism is contraindicated during pregnancy.
B.   Warfarin is excreted in breast milk.
C.   In patients taking warfarin, breastfeeding is contraindicated.
D.   Long-term warfarin therapy may lead to maternal osteoporosis.
E.   Heparin crosses the placenta.
F.   Protamine sulphate is used for heparin overdosage.

82. Haemoglobinopathies:
A.   If both parents are carriers of beta-thalassaemia, the newborn has 1:2 risk of acquiring thalassaemia major.
B.   Alpha-thalassaemia is always due to a deletional defect.
C.   The thalassaemia syndrome is an inherited defect of haemoglobin resulting in a structural abnormality of globin.
D.   HbA (2 alpha 2 beta) should comprise over 50 per cent of the total circulating haemoglobin in the adult.
E.   Sickle-cell haemoglobin is a variant of the alpha globin chain where there is one amino acid substitution at the sixth position.
F.   A patient suffering from sickle-cell anaemia is more likely to be dehydrated during labour.

83. With regards to fetal hydrops:
A.   Hydrops is defined as oedema plus a collection of fluid in at least one visceral cavity.
B.   The incidence of immune hydrops secondary to haemolytic disease is 6:1000 pregnancies.
C.   The approximate incidence of fetal hydrops is 10 per cent of those women with antibodies.
D.   The ratio of non-immune to immune hydrops approximates 2:1.
E.   Non-immune hydrops is defined as the presence of excess extracellular fluid in two or more sites with identifiable circulating antibodies to red blood cell antigens.
F.   Non-immune hydrops is not amenable to intra-uterine therapy.
G.   Non-immune hydrops has a mortality rate of 20–30 per cent.

84. Intrahepatic cholestasis of pregnancy:
A.   Is associated with obstetric haemorrhage.
B.   Proceeds to chronic liver disease in most of cases after delivery.
C.   Jaundice is an essential feature to diagnose.
D.   The recurrence rate in future pregnancy not more than 2 per cent.
E.   May occur in association with oestrogen-containing oral contraceptive.

85. Breast disease:

A. A breast lump with irregular margins is usually benign.
B. A newly diagnosed lump is more likely to be malignant in a 75-year-old woman than in a 30-year-old woman.
C. A normal mammogram in a woman with a palpable mass excludes the diagnosis of malignancy.
D. In mammography, the false-negative rate is thought to be as high as 16 per cent.
E. Tissue histology showing a proliferative pattern is associated with increased risk of malignancy.
F. Breast cysts are more likely to be malignant if the aspirate is blood-stained.

86. Hypertensive disorders in pregnancy:

A. Oedema is present in up to 80 per cent of pregnancies.
B. The serum uric acid concentrations have been found to correlate inversely with renal blood flow per square metre of body surface area.

87. Neurological disease and pregnancy:

A. The anticonvulsant drug sodium valproate does not result in deficiency of vitamin K-dependent clotting factors in the infant.
B. Myotonic dystrophy is exacerbated by pregnancy.
C. A fetus affected by myotonic dystrophy may be identified by oligohydramnios.

88. Causes of non-immune hydrops:

A. Anaemia is the commonest reason for the development of non-immune hydrops.
B. Infective agents can cause the development of non-immune hydrops.
C. 10–20 per cent of cases of non-immune hydrops are associated with chromosomal anomalies.
D. With the help of pre-natal and post-natal tests, a cause can be found in the majority of cases.

89. Puberty:

A. The first sign is the onset of menstruation.
B. Pubertal changes are completed faster in girls than in boys.
C. Growth as measured by height stops at menarche.
D. McCune–Albright syndrome involves delayed pubertal changes.

90. HELLP (haemolysis, elevated liver enzyme, low platelet) syndrome:

A. Describes haemolysis, elevated liver function tests and a low plasma volume.
B. Occurs in 30 per cent of patients with severe pre-eclampsia.
C. Complicates eclampsia in 30 per cent of cases.

91. Auto-immune disease and pregnancy:

A. Systemic lupus erythematosus (SLE): exacerbation during pregnancy may exhibit renal changes indistinguishable from pre-eclampsia.
B. Rheumatoid arthritis (RA) dramatically improves during pregnancy.
C. Patients with RA are less likely to conceive.

92. Transvaginal ultrasound:
A.   Compared with transabdominal scanning specific features of development of the embryo are seen approximately one week earlier.
B.   Is best performed with an empty bladder.
C.   Latex sensitivity is a significant hazard.
D.   The dilated internal cervical os has been demonstrated to be the single most important factor for the prediction of preterm labour.

93. Neonatal lupus erythematosus (NLE) is associated with:
A.   Acquired heart block.
B.   Endocardial fibroelastosis.
C.   Thrombocytopenia.
D.   Aplastic anaemia.
E.   Hepatosplenomegaly.

94. Early pregnancy loss:
A.   Is the commonest medical complication in humans.
B.   Accounts for approximately 75 per cent of emergency gynaecological admissions.
C.   Once a gestational sac has been documented on scan, subsequent loss of viability in the embryonic period is still 11.5 per cent.
D.   The echogenicity of the placenta has been proposed as a sonographic factor associated with early miscarriage.
E.   The volume of a haematoma is a more important prognostic indicator than the site.

95. Magnesium sulphate and eclampsia:
A.   Used properly prevents all seizure activity.
B.   Oral administration is the route of choice.
C.   A loading dose of 40 mg is recommended.
D.   Loss of deep tendon reflexes indicates the need for further magnesium sulphate.
E.   Acts by relieving cerebral vasospasm.

96. Infections and pregnancy:
A.   In affected mothers, vertical transmission of HIV is more common than vertical transmission of syphilis.
B.   Topical treatment of bacterial vaginosis in pregnancy reduces the risk of preterm labour.

97. Group B haemolytic *Streptococcus* (GBS) and the fetus:
A.   Colonized women are at increased risk of premature delivery and perinatal transmission.
B.   GBS is a leading cause of chorioamnionitis and premature rupture of membranes at less than 32 weeks' gestation.
C.   Amniotic infection may cause intra-uterine death.

98. Causes of amenorrhoea include:
A. Gonadal failure.
B. Pregnancy.
C. Metoclopramide.

99. The following relate to double and ectopic ureters:
A. Complete or partial duplication of the ureter results from late splitting of the ureteric bud.
B. With double ureters, the kidneys are usually completely separate.
C. An ectopic ureter may open into the trigone.
D. Ectopic ureters opening below the urethral sphincter do not usually give any clinical or anatomical symptoms.
E. They can be diagnosed prenatally.

100. Varicella zoster:
A. Is a RNA virus of the herpes family.
B. The incubation period is 10–20 days.
C. Is infectious 48 h after the rash appears until the vesicles crust over.
D. Occurs in 1 in 2000 pregnancies.
E. When reactivated as herpes zoster (shingles) does not usually result in intra-uterine infection.
F. Transplacental passage of the virus decreases as gestation advances.
G. If maternal infection occurs 4 days before delivery and up to 2 days postpartum, the infection is lethal in 20–30 per cent of infants.

101. Colposcopy:
A. The aim is to identify the transformation zone of the cervix.
B. Lugol's iodine stains protein within cervical epithelial cells.
C. Increased intercapillary distance is associated with cervical malignancy.

102. The antiphospholipid syndrome:
A. The primary antiphospholipid syndrome (PAPS) refers to the association between second-trimester loss and thrombosis with antiphospholipid antibodies (aPL).
B. Patients with a history of recurrent miscarriage and antiphospholipid antibodies have only a 10 per cent live birth rate in future pregnancies without treatment.
C. Antiphospholipid antibodies interfere with prostacyclin metabolism.

103. Ovarian hyperstimulation syndrome:
A. Gonadotrophin injections are associated with increased risk of ovarian hyperstimulation and multiple pregnancies when used in the treatment of infertility.
B. The risk of ovarian hyperstimulation is 0.6 to 14 per cent of IVF cycles treated with gonadotrophin injections.
C. Ovarian hyperstimulation syndrome is characterized by impaired coagulation.
D. Affected patients should be considered for thromboprophylaxis.

104. Abnormalities of glucose metabolism:
A. The threshold recommended by the WHO to define impaired glucose tolerance (IGT) is a fasting glucose ≥7.8 mmol/L.
B. Using the WHO definition, approximately 1 per cent of apparently normal women in the third trimester will have IGT.
C. IGT in pregnancy is associated with a 50 per cent chance of the woman developing diabetes mellitus in the long term.
D. IGT is not associated with an increased risk of intra-uterine death.
E. The best screening test for IGT is the 50-g glucose load given without dietary preparation.

105. Male factor infertility:
A. Cystic fibrosis may be the reason for male infertility.
B. Asthenospermia means abnormal morphology of sperm.

106. The following conditions are aggravated by pregnancy:
A. Sarcoidosis.
B. Scleroderma.
C. Portal hypertension.
D. Neurofibromatosis.
E. Hodgkin's disease.

107. Perimenopausal women may have dysfunctional uterine bleeding, but endometrial sampling is required to rule out organic disease:
A. Biopsies show endometrial cancer in 2 per cent of cases.
B. Biopsies show normal endometrium in more than 50 per cent of cases.
C. Biopsies show polyps in less than 15 per cent of cases.
D. Biopsies show endometrial hyperplasia in 10–15 per cent of cases.
E. Biopsies show other pathology in 30 per cent of cases.

108. The occlusive diaphragm:
A. Should be used with at least 5 cm (2 inches) of contraceptive cream.
B. Can be used for contraceptive purposes without contraceptive cream or jelly.
C. May be particularly beneficial for prostitutes.
D. The contraceptive diaphragm is available in sizes from 80 to 140 mm diameter.

109. Proteinuria:
A. The average 24-h urinary excretion of protein in non-pregnant subjects is 18 mg.
B. In pregnancy, protein excretion up to 300 mg per 24 h is within normal limits.
C. Reagent strips to test for proteinuria may give a false-negative result if the urine is alkaline.
D. A reading of 2+ on reagent strips corresponds to 1+ g of protein per litre.
E. In patients with pre-eclampsia, proteinuria is significant if there is more than 500 mg in a 24-h urine collection.

110. Chronic hypertension and pregnancy:
A. Is associated with an increased risk of placental abruption.
B. Polyhydramnios is a recognized complication.
C. Anti-hypertensives should be continued even if blood pressure drops to a normal value in the second trimester.
D. There is an increased risk of complications due to intra-uterine growth restriction.

111. With reference to human fertility, the following definitions are correct:
A. The natural fecundity rate is the chance per cycle of becoming pregnant.
B. The normal fecundity rate is about 0.2, or 20 per cent.
C. Infertility is defined as failure to conceive after 1 year of unprotected intercourse.
D. A sperm count of $>20\times10^{6}$/mL is normal.
E. So-called normal semen analysis shows a sperm motility of more than 50 per cent.

112. Calcium metabolism and pregnancy:
A. Approximately 32 g of calcium are passed from mother to fetus during pregnancy.
B. Maternal ionized calcium is decreased in pregnancy.
C. The fetus is hypercalcaemic relative to the mother.

113. Regarding the diagnosis of lichen sclerosis:
A. The diagnosis is histological.
B. It has an atrophic histological appearance.
C. There is thinning atrophy of the epidermis.
D. There is hyalinization of the dermis.
E. There is a subdermal leukocyte infiltration.

114. Ovarian pathology:
A. 80 per cent of ovarian tumours are benign.
B. In polycystic ovary syndrome, follicular cysts are usually large and solitary.
C. Serum Ca125 levels are elevated in patients suffering from endometriosis.
D. Ovarian torsion occurs more often in the right adnexum compared to the left.
E. Most cases of adnexal mass torsion occur in the menopausal years.

115. Oocyte development and ovulation:
A. Primordial follicles represent oocytes arrested within the first meiotic prophase.
B. Ovulation results in extrusion of the first polar body.
C. Ovulation occurs 36 h after the peak of the luteinizing hormone (LH) surge.
D. Prostaglandin levels are maximal just after ovulation.

116. Postnatal morbidity: perineal pain:
A. Occurs in 90 per cent of women after delivery.
B. 10 per cent will have long-term pain 3–18 months after delivery.
C. Ultrasound is a useful treatment modality.

117. Bone metabolism:
A. The bone response to pregnancy is biphasic with early resorption and later bone formation.
B. Cortical bone (hip-like) is more affected by pregnancy than trabecular bone (spine-like).
C. Cortical bone (hip-like) is less affected by heparin than trabecular bone (spine-like).
D. Breast-feeding mothers lose 6 per cent of bone mineral density after 6 months.

118. With regards to electronic fetal monitoring (EFM):
A. Continuous EFM is mandatory during labour.
B. Application of a fetal scalp electrode is atraumatic.

119. Maternal serum alpha-feto protein (MSAFP):
A. A decreased mid-pregnancy level is linked to intra-uterine growth restriction.
B. High levels are associated with subsequent diminished adhesiveness of the placenta.
C. High mid-pregnancy levels in the absence of fetal structural abnormality indicate a decreased risk of placental abruption.

120. Cervical smears:
A. The presence of endocervical cells indicates an inadequate sample.
B. Are immersed in 0.95 per cent ethyl alcohol in order to reduce drying artefact.
C. Human papillomavirus effects and mild dyskaryosis are easily distinguishable.

121. Medical treatment of hirsutism:
A. Cyproterone acetate (CPA) is an effective anti-androgen, which binds to the dihydrotestosterone receptor.
B. The combination of ethinyl oestradiol (EE) and CPA is marketed as Dianette and contains 50 micrograms of EE and 1 mg of CPA.
C. Dianette can be made more potent by the addition of CPA 25–50 mg/day for the first 10 days of each packet.
D. Additional contraception must be used in patients on Dianette because of the risk of feminizing a male fetus.
E. Treatment of hirsutism should be continued for at least 6 months.

122. Regarding polycystic ovarian disease (PCOD):
A. Is exactly the same condition as Stein–Leventhal syndrome.
B. The cysts in PCOD are atretic follicles.
C. Inherited PCOD is transmitted in an autosomal recessive fashion.
D. PCOD is transmitted in an autosomal recessive fashion.
E. The luteinizing hormone:follicle-stimulating hormone (LH: FSH) ratio is decreased in PCOD.
F. The LH: FSH ratio is increased in PCOD.
G. PCOD is characterized by elevated levels of LH.
H. There is a hypersecretion of LH from the posterior pituitary relative to FSH.
I. The mode of inheritance is the same as insulin-dependent diabetes mellitus.
J. Over 90 per cent of patients are oestrogenized.

123. Concerning the antenatal fetal cardiotocograph (CTG):

A. Acceleration is defined as an increase in the fetal heart rate (FHR) of 15 beats per minute (bpm) lasting for at least 30 s.
B. Any deceleration whose lowest point occurs more than 15 s after the peak of the contraction is described as 'late'.
C. Variable decelerations are commonly seen where the umbilical cord is compressed or entangled.

124. Complications of twin pregnancy:

A. In twin-to-twin transfusion syndrome, the haemoglobin levels for both twins are often not discordant.
B. In a twin pregnancy with one fetal loss in the third trimester, in 90 per cent of cases the remaining twin will be delivered within 72 h.
C. Twin reversed arterial perfusion sequence is associated with high mortality in the recipient twin due to prematurity and intra-uterine cardiac failure.
D. With significant growth discordance, particularly when the first twin is the smaller, Caesarean section is the preferred route of delivery.

125. Antepartum haemorrhage (APH):

A. Is defined as bleeding from the genital tract after 24 weeks' gestation.
B. If associated with labour-like pains, a vaginal examination is advisable.
C. In cases of placental abruption, there is coincident placenta praevia in 1 per cent of patients.

126. Physiology of pregnancy:

A. Dyspnoea is an uncommon complication of pregnancy.
B. Cardiac output increases immediately after delivery.
C. Heart murmurs are a common finding in pregnancy.
D. No change in plasma volume occurs before 20 weeks' gestation.

127. Termination of pregnancy:

A. The 1967 Abortion Act legalized abortion in England, Scotland, Wales and Northern Ireland.
B. Is available 'on demand' for social reasons up to 24 weeks of pregnancy.
C. Since the 1990 Human Fertilisation and Embryo Act, it may be performed at any gestation if severe fetal abnormality is detected.
D. The 'blue form' (the statutory form to be completed prior to any termination of pregnancy) needs to be signed by three independent medical doctors.

128. ICSI (intracytoplasmic sperm injection):

A. Is only successful if the whole sperm is injected into an oocyte.
B. Successfully overcomes azoospermia associated with obstruction.

129. Concerning the spread of endometrial carcinoma:

A. A minority of cases have penetrated the myometrium by more than two-thirds at diagnosis.
B. Myometrial invasion correlates well with tumour grade.
C. Lymph node metastases are found in more than 50 per cent of cases.
D. Metastases in the ovary are common.
E. The presence of tumour in areas of adenomyosis confers a poor prognosis.

130. Placental abruption:

A. Is defined as the premature separation of an abnormally sited placenta.
B. 70–80 per cent result in vaginal bleeding.
C. The bleeding is typically bright red and clotting.
D. In 50 per cent of cases the bleeding occurs after 36 weeks' gestation.
E. Blood loss is invariably of maternal origin.
F. Tends to recur in subsequent pregnancies.

131. Tamoxifen:

A. In a premenopausal woman, additional contraception is not necessary.
B. May cause spontaneous abortion.
C. Is an oestrogen-receptor antagonist.
D. Has weak oestrogen-like activity.
E. Has no effect on oestrogen receptor-negative tumours.

132. The epidemiology of osteoporosis in the UK:

A. Osteoporosis costs the NHS nearly £1 billion annually.
B. The lifetime incidence of hip fracture in women is 25 per cent.
C. The WHO definition is a T-score below −2.0 on bone mineral density scanning.

133. Placenta praevia:

A. Nulliparity is a risk factor.
B. Complicates approximately 1 in 400 pregnancies.
C. Is associated with intra-uterine growth restriction.
D. Fetal growth restriction is more commonly encountered in association with placenta praevia than with normally sited placentas.
E. Is commonly encountered in those who have previously been delivered by Caesarean section.
F. Four Caesarean section scars increases the risk by more than 50 per cent.
G. Is associated with a maternal mortality rate of 0.3 per cent in the UK.
H. Transvaginal ultrasound is the diagnostic technique of choice.

134. Regarding vaginal delivery:

A. More than 70 per cent of deliveries in the UK require instrumental assistance.
B. Operative vaginal delivery has been directly linked to faecal incontinence.
C. Forceps deliveries and vacuum extractions may be performed before full dilatation of the cervix.

135. Heart disease in pregnancy:

A. Heart disease due to rheumatic fever is the most common cardiac complication of pregnancy in the UK.
B. The number of women with congenital cardiac lesions reaching childbearing age has decreased.
C. The number of maternal deaths due to cardiac disease continues to fall.
D. Severe cardiac disease is a contraindication to ergometrine administration.
E. An intra-uterine contraceptive device (IUCD) is the contraceptive method of choice for the patient with valvular heart disease.
F. Beta-blocking drugs are contraindicated in the pregnant patient.
G. In Eisenmenger's complex there is an interatrial septal defect.

136. Abdominal wall defects:

A. Exomphalos is associated with chromosomal abnormalities in 80 per cent of cases.
B. Exomphalos is a synonym for gastroschisis.
C. Gastroschisis is associated with chromosomal abnormalities in 10 per cent of cases.
D. Ectopia vesica is associated with gastroschisis.

137. Pre-eclampsia:

A. Pre-eclampsia consists of a diagnostic triad of elevated blood pressure, proteinuria and oedema.
B. Chronic hypertension and pre-eclampsia cannot co-exist.
C. Pre-eclampsia occurs in 50 per cent of pregnancies.
D. Severe pre-eclampsia is characterized by raised blood pressure in association with proteinuria of at least 5 g per 24 h.
E. The cause of pre-eclampsia remains unclear.
F. Smoking is a risk factor for pre-eclampsia.

138. Hyperemesis gravidarum:

A. Urinary tract infection is the commonest cause of vomiting in the first trimester.
B. Steroids are contraindicated in the treatment of intractable vomiting in pregnancy.
C. Is associated with tetany.
D. Is associated with cerebellar ataxia.

139. Regarding mode of delivery:

A. Maternal mortality after Caesarean section is no higher than after vaginal delivery.
B. There is no role for prophylactic antibiotics at the time of Caesarean section.
C. Vacuum delivery results in less maternal morbidity than forceps delivery.
D. The use of a vacuum extractor compared to forceps is associated with fewer cases of cephalhaematoma.
E. The use of a vacuum extractor compared to forceps results in significantly better Apgar scores.

140. Lichen sclerosis:
A. Is mainly a condition of post-menopausal women.
B. The classical appearance is of a red, thickened vulva with shiny, papery skin on the vulva extending to encircle the anus in a figure-of-eight fashion.
C. Involutional adhesion of the labia minora to the labia majora is a characteristic feature.
D. In the male it is called 'balanitis xerotica obliterans'.
E. Affects only vaginal skin.
F. Less than 5 per cent of lesions occur in non-genital skin.
G. The risk of progression to invasive carcinoma is 30–40 per cent.

141. Risk factors for endometrial carcinoma associated with postmenopausal bleeding include:
A. Nulliparity.
B. Early menopause.
C. Use of the combined oral contraceptive pill (COCP).
D. Hypertension.
E. Use of the intra-uterine contraceptive device (IUCD).

142. Postpartum endometritis:
A. The most common infective agent causing pelvic infection in the postpartum period is *Staphylococcus aureus*.
B. The majority of infected patients have asymptomatic cervical infection.
C. The incidence of death due to genital tract sepsis has increased in recent years.

143. Adverse effects of the intra-uterine contraceptive device (IUCD):
A. 1 per cent of nulliparous patients will develop tubal occlusion.
B. The rate of uterine perforation is 3–6 per 1000 during insertion.

144. Recognized complications of diagnostic hysteroscopy:
A. Perforation.
B. Water intoxication.
C. Pulmonary oedema.
D. Air embolism.
E. Anaphylaxis.

145. Irritable bowel syndrome (IBS):
A. Is a functional bowel disorder.
B. Is a physical bowel disorder.
C. Affects about 20 per cent of all people at any one time.
D. May be characterized by sigmoid tenderness.
E. May be improved by psychotherapy.
F. Defaecation exacerbates the pain.

146. Regarding vaginal breech delivery:
A. Arrest of the after coming head occurs in 50 per cent of cases.
B. Hypoxia is an uncommon cause of perinatal mortality.
C. Hyperextension of the neck is associated with trisomy 21.
D. Artificial rupture of the membranes is recommended in the early stages of labour.
E. Respiratory distress is less common in babies born by Caesarean section.

147. Sex chromosome abnormalities:
A. The incidence of Turner's syndrome (XO) rises with maternal age.
B. Turner's syndrome is lethal in over 95 per cent of cases.
C. Cystic hygroma is associated with Turner's syndrome.
D. All cases of Turner's syndrome (XO) are due to a gene deletion.
E. Occur with the same frequency as autosomal abnormalities in livebirths.
F. Offspring of parents with XXX syndrome are at a higher risk of premature menopause.
G. The incidence of XXY (Klinefelter's syndrome) is decreased with advanced maternal age.
H. The XXY male is characteristically tall, with gynaecomastia.
I. The XXY male has a normal sperm count, but is infertile due to hypoplasia of the vas deferens.
J. The incidence of XXXX syndrome is increased in offspring of beer drinkers in Australia.

148. The following statements are true about endometrial carcinoma:
A. It is seen most commonly in the 65- to 75-year age group.
B. It is very rare in women under the age of 40 years.
C. It is more aggressive in postmenopausal women.
D. It is frequently seen in cases of untreated Turner's syndrome.
E. It is related to polycystic ovary syndrome.

149. Thromboembolic disease:
A. Thromboembolic disease in pregnancy remains the commonest cause of maternal death and has a 10 per cent recurrence risk.
B. Venography and isotope lung scans are contraindicated during pregnancy for the diagnosis of thromboembolic disease.
C. Treatment of thromboembolic disease in pregnancy with subcutaneous heparin may cause thrombocytopenia.

150. Premenstrual syndrome (PMS):
A. Is more common in multiparous patients.
B. To diagnose PMS, the symptoms must be present for four out of five cycles.

151. Shoulder dystocia:

A. Occurs when the fetal shoulders present an excessive diameter to the maternal pelvic inlet.
B. Complicates 50 per cent of deliveries.
C. Never occurs in babies weighing <4 kg.
D. McRoberts manoeuvre involves marked extension of the maternal hips.
E. Brachial plexus injury is most often due to clavicular fractures.
F. Suprapubic pressure and correct positioning of legs with an adequate episiotomy facilitates delivery of 10 per cent of cases of shoulder dystocia.
G. The incidence is increased in infants of diabetic mothers.
H. Maternal diabetes mellitus increases the risk of shoulder dystocia to 70 per cent.

152. The puerperium:

A. Refers to the first 6 months after delivery.
B. Problems arising in the puerperium become chronic in more than 40 per cent of patients.
C. The lochia usually persists for 7 weeks.
D. The uterine fundus should not be palpable abdominally 14 days after delivery.
E. Anaemia occurs in 25–30 per cent of patients.
F. The incidence of postnatal depression is 50 per cent.

153. Features of testicular feminization include:

A. Primary amenorrhoea.
B. Normal breast development.
C. Absence of a uterus.

154. Gestational trophoblastic disease:

A. A gestational trophoblastic tumour cannot occur after a normal pregnancy.
B. A gestational trophoblastic tumour occurring after a full-term pregnancy is always choriocarcinoma.
C. The incidence of choriocarcinoma following a complete mole is of the order of 3 per cent.
D. Persistent postpartum haemorrhage may be a sign of gestational trophoblastic tumour.
E. After 12 months of remission from gestational trophoblastic tumour, there is no contraindication to pregnancy.

155. Mifepristone:

A. Is a synthetic progesterone agonist derived from norethisterone.
B. Is licensed for medical termination up to 12 weeks' gestation.
C. When combined with gemeprost, will result in 99 per cent of pregnancies aborting in the first trimester.

156. The following are recognized causes of urinary incontinence:
A. Overflow incontinence.
B. Immobility.
C. Urethral diverticulae.
D. Urinary tract infection.
E. Faecal impaction.

157. Regarding milk synthesis:
A. Serum prolactin levels are constant during the first week of the postnatal period.
B. Prolactin acts directly to stimulate milk synthesis.
C. Human milk contains more sodium than cows' milk.

158. Tamoxifen actions include:
A. A decrease in the number of progesterone receptors.
B. An oestrogen-like maintenance of bone.
C. A significant increase in thrombotic events.
D. Increased risk of hepatic carcinoma with very large doses.
E. An improvement in endometriosis.

159. In preterm premature rupture of the membranes (PROM):
A. The risk to the fetus is directly proportional to the gestational age.
B. There is an increased risk of placental abruption.
C. At a gestational age less than 28 weeks, it is seldom treated conservatively.
D. Vaginal examinations should be avoided in all cases.
E. If chorioamnionitis is suspected, the most appropriate antibiotic is a cephalosporin.
F. Histological chorioamnionitis is found in 42–85 per cent of cases.

160. Urethral caruncle:
A. Is associated with chronic trichomonas infection and may recur after surgical treatment.
B. May cause urge incontinence.
C. Is treated by excision biopsy.
D. Is rarely found on the posterior aspect of the external urethral meatus.
E. Is a premalignant lesion.

161. Breast problems:
A. The most common problem in the puerperium is breast tenderness.
B. Breast abscesses are more common in the first week of the postpartum period than in the second.
C. In the presence of mastitis, breast-feeding mothers should be advised to discontinue feeds from the affected side.

162. Thromboembolic disease:
A. Is the commonest cause of direct maternal death.
B. The risk of developing a venous thromboembolism increases with maternal age.

163. Episiotomy:
A. Routine episiotomy is recommended for all vaginal deliveries in the UK.
B. Rectal extensions are more common with mediolateral episiotomies.
C. It has been clearly shown that routine episiotomy is an effective preventative measure against third- and fourth-degree tears.

164. Burch colposuspension:
A. Enterocele formation occurs postoperatively in up to 18 per cent of patients.
B. The incidence of de-novo detrusor instability is 18 per cent.
C. If preoperative urodynamic assessment shows a reduced peak urinary flow rate of <15 mL/s or a maximum voiding pressure of 15 cm H_2O, then Burch colposuspension should be avoided.
D. Cure rates are improved if abdominal hysterectomy is performed at the same time.

165. Gestational diabetes mellitus (GDM):
A. May only be diagnosed when insulin therapy is required.
B. Is impossible to distinguish from overt diabetes mellitus type I.
C. Is associated with an increased risk of congenital malformations.

166. Trophoblastic disease:
A. The most common chromosomal pattern of a complete mole is 46XY.
B. In complete mole the chromosomal pattern is paternally derived.
C. Embryonic tissue is often present in complete moles.
D. The chromosomal pattern with a partial mole is diploid.
E. In cases of partial mole, the fetus never survives to term.

167. The following are true statements about fetal pain:
A. The fetus can feel pain before 22 weeks' gestation.
B. Analgesia is needed during termination of pregnancy for any fetus greater than 24 weeks' gestation.

168. Urge incontinence:
A. Psychotherapy (e.g. biofeedback, hypnotherapy and acupuncture) has a high success rate.
B. Urinalysis and urine culture and sensitivity are essential investigations.
C. May be caused by multiple sclerosis.

169. Classification of episiotomies:
A. Extension of an episiotomy into the rectal mucosa is classified as a third-degree tear.
B. Second-degree tears involve partial or complete disruption of the anal sphincter.
C. Fourth-degree tears involve partial or complete disruption of the anal sphincter only.

170. The following statements are true about placenta praevia:

A. Transabdominal ultrasound (TAS) has a false-positive rate of 20 per cent for the diagnosis of placenta praevia.
B. An overdistended maternal bladder makes the diagnosis easier by (TAS).
C. The diagnostic accuracy of transvaginal ultrasound (TVS) is greater than abdominal ultrasound.
D. TAS has a diagnostic accuracy of 93–97 per cent.
E. Only 5 per cent of patients diagnosed as having a low-lying placenta in the second trimester continue to have placenta praevia at delivery.

171. Thromboembolic disease in pregnancy:

A. 90 per cent of patients with pulmonary embolism are diagnosed correctly on a clinical basis.
B. High parity is a risk factor for developing thromboembolic disease.
C. A woman with a history of venous thromboembolism in a previous pregnancy needs anticoagulant medication throughout subsequent pregnancies.
D. Emergency Caesarean section is a risk factor for venous thromboembolism, and must be treated with heparin prophylaxis in the postoperative period.
E. Elective Caesarean section is an absolute indication for thromboprophylaxis with heparin.
F. Patients with antiphospholipid antibody are at high risk of developing venous thromboembolism in labour.

172. Anticoagulation:

A. Low molecular-weight heparins are the drug of choice to treat venous thromboembolism in the antenatal period.
B. Full anticoagulation with warfarin is a contraindication to epidural anaesthesia.
C. Osteosclerosis is a recognized side effect of heparin use in pregnancy.
D. The standard prophylactic dose of unfractionated heparin is 50 000 IU twice daily, subcutaneously.

173. Breast cancer:

A. There is evidence that the risk of breast cancer is increased after pregnancy.
B. Pregnant women who develop breast cancer soon after pregnancy have the same prognosis as non-pregnant women.
C. Women who develop breast cancer during or soon after pregnancy would be expected to have bigger tumours.
D. Up to 50 per cent of women who are fertile after treatment for breast cancer will go on to have children.
E. The 10-year survival rate of patients who have pregnancies after having breast cancer is less than 10 per cent.
F. Pregnancy after breast cancer treatment should be delayed for at least 5 years.
G. Breast-feeding is contraindicated for patients who have had conservative management of breast cancer.
H. Termination of pregnancy does not change the overall survival rate.

174. Auto-immune disease:
A. Most auto-immune diseases occur in women of childbearing age.
B. Lupus anticoagulant and anticardiolipin antibodies are both classified as antiphospholipid antibodies.
C. Antiphospholipid antibodies are not associated with recurrent miscarriage.
D. In patients experiencing recurrent miscarriage (three consecutive losses), more than 50 per cent show clinically relevant levels of antiphospholipid antibodies.
E. Lupus anticoagulant is associated with decreased tendency to clot.
F. More than 70 per cent of patients with lupus anticoagulant have anticardiolipin antibodies.
G. Antiphospholipid syndrome is diagnosed on laboratory findings only.
H. Studies show low-dose aspirin therapy to be beneficial to pregnant patients with antiphospholipid syndrome.

175. The following are complications of fibroids in pregnancy:
A. Malpresentation.
B. Placenta accreta.
C. Placenta praevia.
D. Necrobiosis.

176. Haematological disorders:
A. Haematuria and fat embolism are recognized features of sickle-cell disease in pregnancy.
B. Patients with sickle-cell anaemia have a lower incidence of thromboembolic disease.
C. If both parents are carriers of beta-thalassaemia, the newborn has 50 per cent chance of acquiring thalassaemia major.

177. Aspirin:
A. Inhibits thromboxane synthesis by platelets.
B. The CLASP trial showed a significant reduction in pre-eclampsia in patients treated with aspirin 60 mg daily from 12 weeks.
C. Low-dose aspirin taken before 16 weeks' gestation reduced the risks of early-onset pre-eclampsia (PET) (<32 weeks).

178. Fibroids:
A. Fibroids are benign tumours of striated muscle.
B. Have the highest incidence in the seventh decade of life.
C. Grow in response to the combined oral contraceptive pill.
D. Submucosal fibroids lie just below the endometrium.
E. 20 per cent of fibroids contain malignant tissue.
F. May extend directly into the heart.
G. Never occur on the vulva.
H. Submucous fibroids project from the peritoneal surface of the uterus.
I. Parasitic fibroids are pedunculated fibroids, which lose their uterine attachment and gain a secondary blood supply.
J. Fibroids found at Caesarean section should be removed.
K. After myomectomy, any subsequent pregnancy should be delivered by Caesarean section.
L. Ovarian failure is a recognized complication after radiological embolization.

179. The following features indicate heart disease in pregnancy:
A. The presence of a third heart sound.
B. The apex beat is palpable in the axilla.
C. An early diastolic murmur.

180. Epilepsy:
A. In the epileptic pregnant woman there is an increased risk of placental abruption.
B. Women planning pregnancy, on drug treatment for epilepsy, should take a daily dose of 15 mg folic acid.
C. The risk of a fetus being born with epilepsy for an epileptic mother is 1:80.
D. Carbamazepine may cause neonatal bleeding.
E. The pregnant mother taking phenytoin should be given vitamin K before delivery.
F. Migraine, rheumatoid arthritis and epilepsy tend to improve with pregnancy.

181. Physiotherapy:
A. Can cure or improve 75 per cent of patients with genuine stress incontinence (GSI).
B. 5 years after a successful course of physiotherapy 75 per cent of women remain cured.
C. A frequency of 10 Hz (hertz) is used during electrostimulation of fast muscle fibres.
D. A success rate of up to 90 per cent can be achieved by pelvic floor exercises in the conservative management of GSI.

182. Ovarian germ cell tumours:
A. The majority are malignant.
B. The most common malignant germ cell tumour is a dysgerminoma.
C. Premenarchal patients should undergo karyotyping.
D. Human chorionic gonadotrophin (hCG) and lactate dehydrogenase (LDH) are useful tumour markers.
E. Dysgerminomas are almost always bilateral.

183. Pre-eclampsia:
A. Is associated with acute arterial atherosis.
B. Is associated with glomerular endotheliosis.
C. Is associated with lack of trophoblast infiltration of arterial wall.
D. Is associated with decreased arterial sensitivity to angiotensin II.
E. Is most likely inherited as a single dominant trait.
F. Is more common in monozygotic than dizygotic twins.
G. Phenytoin is the anticonvulsant of choice in severe pre-eclampsia.
H. Severe pre-eclampsia can result in liver failure, thrombocytopenia and blindness.

184. Obstetric perineal trauma:
A. 10 per cent of women who have a vaginal birth also sustain some degree of perineal trauma.
B. Anterior perineal trauma includes injury to labia, vagina, urethra, clitoris and bladder.
C. Inability to control flatus after vaginal delivery is attributed to nerve damage alone.

185. Hydatidiform mole:
A. If serum levels of serum beta hCG fall to normal within 70 days, follow-up is limited to 6 months.
B. Chemotherapy is required if the serum human chorionic gonadotrophin (hCG) level is more than 10 000 IU/L at 4 weeks after evacuation of the mole.
C. Hormonal contraception can be taken as soon as serum hCG level falls to normal.
D. hCG levels should be checked after any future normal pregnancy.
E. Some patients require 2-year follow-up. Once hCG level has been normal for more than 6 months, there is no risk of choriocarcinoma developing.

186. Thromboprophylaxis in gynaecology:
A. Thromboembolic disease accounts for 20 per cent of perioperative deaths in gynaecology.
B. The risk of postoperative thromboembolism in users of the low-dose pill is estimated to be twice that of non-users.
C. Hormone replacement therapy (HRT) should be stopped prior to surgery because of its association with venous thromboembolism.

187. Physical properties of ultrasound:
A. The American Institute of Ultrasound in Medicine (AIUM) advises that there is no risk of damaging tissue through heating as long as the 'thermal index' score (TIS) is kept lower than 20.
B. The lateral extent of the Field of View is determined by the Sector Angle that the beam sweeps through.
C. When using a modern ultrasound scanner, a higher frequency will give better resolution.
D. When using a modern ultrasound scanner, a higher frequency will give deeper penetration.

188. Side effects of hormone replacement therapy (HRT): continuous combined therapy and breakthrough bleeding (BTB):
A. Occurs in 40–60 per cent of patients during the first 6 months of treatment.
B. Occurs in 20 per cent after the first year.
C. Is similar in mechanism to that seen with oral contraceptives.
D. May require a change to a sequential programme if it persists beyond 1 year.
E. Can be stopped by the addition of a higher dose of progestin.

189. Postnatal morbidity-stress incontinence:
A. Approximately 20 per cent of women suffer stress incontinence for the first time after delivery.
B. Approximately 50 per cent of women will suffer from stress incontinence 3 months after delivery.
C. Postnatal exercises are excellent prophylactic measures against stress incontinence in the postnatal period.
D. Approximately 5 per cent of women will experience de-novo urinary frequency after delivery.

190. First-trimester miscarriage:

A. About 20 per cent of women will experience first-trimester vaginal bleeding.
B. Serum beta human chorionic gonadotrophin (hCG) levels double every 48 h in a patient with incomplete miscarriage.
C. After a complete miscarriage, serum beta hCG levels return to normal within 24 h.
D. Monoclonal antibody tests can detect hCG at a concentration of 1 IU/L.
E. The administration of exogenous progesterone in early pregnancy does not prevent miscarriage.

191. Risk factors for cervical cancer include:

A. First coitus at a young age.
B. Single sexual partner.
C. Lower socioeconomic status.
D. Human papillomavirus (HPV).

192. The third stage of labour:

A. The routine use of oxytocics has been shown to improve haemoglobin levels.
B. Ergometrine should be routinely used in all patients in the third stage.
C. Ergometrine may be used safely in management of the third stage of labour for a hypertensive patient.
D. The incidence of retained placenta after vaginal delivery is 2 per cent.
E. Waiting 60 min rather than 30 min will halve the number of women requiring an anaesthetic for manual removal of the placenta.

193. Detrusor instability:

A. May be improved by low-frequency neuromuscular electrical stimulation (NMS).
B. May be improved by psychotherapy.
C. May be improved by TENS (transcutaneous electrical nerve stimulation).
D. May be improved by S3 sacral nerve stimulation.
E. May be improved by distigmine bromide.

194. In endometrial carcinoma, the histological subtype:

A. Is endometrioid in 30 per cent of cases.
B. Is endometrioid with squamous differentiation in 25 per cent of cases.
C. Is clear cell adenocarcinoma in fewer than 10 per cent of cases.
D. Mucinous adenocarcinoma and squamous cell carcinoma are rare findings.
E. Should contain more than 10 per cent of a second pattern to be classified as mixed carcinoma.

195. Ovulation:
A. Clomiphene citrate is the most common drug used to induce ovulation.
B. Clomiphene citrate blocks oestrogen receptors in the ovary.
C. Patients treated with clomiphene citrate have a 5–10 per cent chance of multiple pregnancy.
D. Dexamethasone can be used in treatment of anovulation.
E. Strenuous exercise may result in anovulation due to decreased amplitude of gonadotrophin-releasing hormone (GnRH) excretion.
F. The ovaries of young women cannot fail to respond to stimulation by pituitary gonadotrophins.
G. Clomiphene citrate can be used in women with normal prolactin and gonadotrophin levels.
H. Wedge resection of ovaries is considered first-line treatment in anovulation associated with polycystic ovarian disease.
I. Treatment of ovarian disorders is more successful than treatment of other causes of infertility with respect to pregnancy.

196. Regarding perineal massage:
A. When practised in labour it does not protect against the trauma of delivery.
B. When conducted antenatally it does not protect against the trauma of delivery.
C. Should be prohibited in labour as it does more harm than good.
D. In the second stage of labour, it reduces the likelihood of dyspareunia at 3 months postpartum.
E. In the second stage of labour, it reduces the likelihood of urinary incontinence.

197. Erectile dysfunction:
A. May be caused by cimetidine (Tagamet).
B. Is usually due to a physical problem.
C. May be treated with sildenafil (Viagra).
D. May be treated with apomorphine.
E. Drug treatment is useful in Peyronie's disease.

198. The combined oral contraceptive pill (COCP):
A. Is relatively safe to continue up to the age of 40 in a woman who smokes.
B. 20–30 per cent of women in their 40s use the COCP.
C. Contains 0.2–0.5 mg of ethinyl oestradiol.
D. Ovulation is prevented by the progestogen.
E. May be less effective in patients with epilepsy on medication.

199. Regarding vulval intraepithelial neoplasia (VIN):
A. VIN II involves the upper two-thirds of the vulvar squamous epithelium.
B. In up to 75 per cent of women, the presenting complaint is pruritus.
C. The majority of lesions involve non-hairy skin exclusively.
D. The most common site affected is the anterior one-third of the inner labia majora.
E. The majority of lesions are unifocal.

200. Chorionic villus sampling (CVS):

A. May be used earlier than amniocentesis to establish a diagnosis (>11 weeks).
B. The miscarriage rate after CVS at 11–14 weeks is the same as that for amniocentesis at 16 weeks.
C. 10 per cent of cultures obtained by CVS will show mosaicism of the placenta.

201. Vaginismus:

A. May be a cause of female sexual dysfunction.
B. Is defined as the voluntary spasm of the muscle surrounding the vaginal outlet.
C. Only occurs in response to an actual attempt at penetration.

202. Non-neoplastic disorders of the vulva (NNDV):

A. Vulval atrophy is always symptomatic.
B. Simple vulvectomy is an effective and permanent treatment for chronic vulval dystrophy.
C. Vulval dystrophy often reappears after such surgery.
D. The classification of vulval disorders (ISSVD 1986) includes 'hyperplastic dystrophy', 'lichen sclerosis' and 'other dermatoses' as non-neoplastic disorders of the vulva.
E. In this classification, Paget's disease is a non-squamous vulval intraepithelial neoplasia (VIN).
F. The finding of adjacent areas of squamous hyperplasia with lichen sclerosis is regarded as part of the spectrum of lichen sclerosis.
G. The pruritus associated with vulval dystrophy is often worse early in the day.
H. Lichen planus may present as a vulval dermatosis.
I. Sarcoidosis can present with symptoms of vulval dystrophy.

203. Pelvic pain:

A. Fibroids are a common cause.
B. Deep vaginal pain post hysterectomy may be demonstrated via trigger points in the vaginal cuff.
C. A history of sexual abuse is associated with chronic pelvic pain.

204. Dysmenorrhoea:

A. Secondary dysmenorrhoea usually precedes menstrual loss.
B. Mefenamic acid acts to relieve dysmenorrhoea by an antifibrinolytic mechanism.

205. Tamoxifen:

A. Is a steroidal compound structurally related to diethylstilboestrol.
B. Competitively inhibits oestrogen binding by binding to the oestrogen receptor.
C. In premenopausal women, it has an anti-oestrogenic effect.
D. In women with breast cancer, there is an increased survival at 5 years of approximately 20 per cent.
E. Is associated with a 2- to 4-fold increased risk of endometrial cancer.

206. Haemorrhagic disease of the newborn (HDN):

A. Can be prevented by prophylactic vitamin K administration to the newborn.
B. Vitamin K administration by the intramuscular route may predispose to childhood leukaemia.

207. Ca125 is elevated (normal range <35 U/mL) in the following conditions:
A. Menstruation.
B. 50 per cent of stage 1 ovarian cancers.
C. Pelvic inflammatory disease.
D. Urinary tract infection.
E. Pancreatic cancer.

208. Maternal serum alpha-fetoprotein (MSAFP) will be raised if the fetus is affected by:
A. Trisomy 21 (Down's syndrome).
B. Trisomy 18 (Edward's syndrome).
C. Open neural tube defect at 16 weeks' gestation.
D. Normal ultrasound scan findings.
E. Intra-uterine death.
F. Rhesus disease.
G. Gastroschisis.
H. Epidermolysis bullosa.

209. Primary dysmenorrhoea:
A. Is pelvic pain in the absence of pelvic disease.
B. Characteristically results in pelvic pain for the week preceding menstrual flow.
C. The level of uterine prostaglandins correlates poorly with severity of menstrual cramps.
D. The combined oral contraceptive pill is an unsuitable treatment.
E. Is exacerbated by caffeine.
F. Usually commences in adult life.

210. Complications of tocolytic therapy:
A. The risks with beta-sympathomimetics are the same in multiple pregnancy as in singleton pregnancy.
B. Beta-sympathomimetics used for tocolysis are associated with hyperglycaemia, hypertension and pyrexia.
C. Include cyanosis and dyspnoea.

211. If the fetal bowel appears echogenic in the mid-trimester:
A. There may be intra-uterine growth retardation.
B. Both parents should be tested for cystic fibrosis.
C. Fetal karyotyping should be performed.
D. It may be a normal ultrasound finding.

212. Postmaturity:
A. Prolonged pregnancy refers to pregnancy lasting more than 294 days from the first day of the last menstrual period.
B. Postmaturity syndrome includes dry peeling skin, well-developed palmar creases and coating of the body with meconium.
C. The incidence of antepartum death, intrapartum death and neonatal death are approximately equal in prolonged pregnancy.

213. Placenta praevia:
A. Complicates approximately 1 in 400 pregnancies.
B. Is associated with a maternal mortality rate of 0.3 per cent in the UK.
C. Transvaginal ultrasound is the diagnostic technique of choice.
D. If the placental edge is less than 3 cm from the internal cervical os, a Caesarean section should be performed.
E. There is a significant association between placenta praevia and placenta accreta.

214. Menorrhagia:
A. Normal menstrual blood loss is 100–150 mL.
B. Occurs more commonly in anovulatory cycles.
C. Endometrial ablation is more successful in the presence of uterine pathology such as fibroids.
D. 40 per cent of patients suffering from menorrhagia with demonstrable pathology have adenomyosis.
E. Adenomyosis may be diagnosed on Pipelle sampling.

215. Dysfunctional uterine bleeding (DUB):
A. Has an easily identifiable cause.
B. Usually occurs in anovulatory cycles.
C. Every patient should undergo hysteroscopy.
D. With anovulation is easier to treat than DUB associated with ovulatory cycles.
E. Progestogen therapy is recommended as a first-line treatment for ovulatory DUB.
F. Patients being treated for DUB with Provera may also assume contraceptive cover.

216. Features of human papillomavirus (HPV) infection in squamous cells:
A. Cytoplasmic vacuolization.
B. Nuclear enlargement.
C. Hyperchromasia.
D. Chromatin clumping.

217. Cervical intraepithelial neoplasia (CIN):
A. Preinvasive lesions of the cervix are more common in patients with two or fewer sexual partners.

218. Bartholin's glands:
A. Secrete mucus.
B. A Bartholin's abscess is equivalent to an infected Bartholin's cyst.
C. All Bartholin's cysts should be excised.
D. Most Bartholin's abscesses contain a mixture of bacterial organisms.
E. Bartholin's cysts are always due to infection.

219. Lymphogranuloma venereum:
A. Is a sexually transmitted disease.
B. Is caused by the Donovan bacillus.
C. Is characterized by inguinal lymphangitis, anogenital lesions and fibrosis.

220. Endometriosis and treatment options:
A. Symptom recurrence following medical treatment is unusual.
B. Laser treatment is more effective than electrocautery.
C. The combined oral contraceptive pill is an ineffective way of managing endometriosis.
D. Elevated Ca125 is associated with patients who benefit from early laparoscopy.
E. Laparoscopic ablation of endometriosis works best in mild/moderate cases.

221. Progesterone-only contraception is ideal for:
A. Diabetics.
B. Hypertensives.

222. Trisomy 21 (Down's syndrome):
A. 95 per cent of cases are due to non-dysjunction.
B. The overall incidence is 1:650 livebirths.
C. Affected children are mildly mentally retarded.
D. Congenital heart disease is common among affected children.
E. Gastro-intestinal tract abnormalities are unusual among affected children.
F. Most affected babies die before the age of one year.

223. Choroid plexus cysts:
A. Are present in 1 per cent of all 20-week normality ultrasound scans.
B. Are often associated with trisomy 21 (Down's syndrome).

224. The following are true regarding cervical carcinoma:
A. Human papillomavirus (HPV) type 16 and 18 are associated with most cervical intracepithelial neoplasia (CIN) lesions of all grades and invasive cancer.
B. Stage IIIb indicates that the carcinoma extends beyond the cervix, but not to the pelvic side wall.
C. 5-year survival for stage Iia is 85–90 per cent, whatever the method used for treatment.

225. Antibiotics and preterm labour:
A. A woman with ruptured membranes at 30 weeks' gestation should be started on antibiotics.
B. Prophylactic antibiotics in women with premature preterm rupture of membranes reduce both maternal and fetal infection.
C. Antibiotic therapy decreases the odds of delivering within 1 week of membrane rupture by about 10 per cent when given to women with ruptured membranes in the absence of uterine activity between 27 and 33 weeks' gestation.

226. Endometriosis and fertility:
A. Over 90 per cent of patients present with fertility problems.
B. Women with endometriosis-associated infertility have a good chance of conception with hormonal treatment.
C. For patients with endometriosis-associated infertility, medical treatment is the best option.
D. Gonadotrophins have no use in the treatment of infertility secondary to endometriosis.

227. Vulval pathology:
A. Vulval cancer is associated with nulliparity.
B. Lichen sclerosis is found adjacent to 30 per cent of vulval cancers.

228. Pelvic congestion syndrome:
A. Deep dyspareunia is a typical symptom.
B. Patients usually complain of a localized suprapubic pain.
C. Medroxyprogesterone acetate has been shown to be a useful treatment.

229. Post-coital contraception (PCC):
A. The combined oral contraceptive pill cannot be used as a form of PCC.
B. Mifepristone produces its action through changes in the tubal epithelium.
C. The PCC dose of levonorgestrel is two 75 mg doses, 12 h apart.
D. Previous thrombosis is the only contraindication to PCC methods containing oestrogen.

230. Cancer of the vulva:
A. May be caused by human papillomavirus (HPV).
B. Is predominantly adencarcinoma.
C. Cloquet's node is the deepest node of the femoral group.
D. Malignant melanoma is the second most common vulval malignancy.
E. Chemotherapy is an effective treatment.

231. Menorrhagia:
A. One in three women will describe heavy menstrual bleeding at some stage in their life.
B. 50 per cent of women who complain of menorrhagia have a measured blood flow within normal limits.
C. Is usually due to an easily identifiable cause.
D. Lifetime risk of hysterectomy is estimated to be 50 per cent.

232. Tranexamic acid:
A. Works by inhibiting fibrinolysis.
B. One-third of women will experience gastro-intestinal side effects with 3–6 g daily.
C. Is associated with an increased risk of deep venous thrombosis.
D. Is better at reducing menstrual blood loss than mefenamic acid.
E. Intracranial thrombosis is a serious side effect.

233. Medical treatment of hyperprolactinoma:
A. Bromocriptine normalizes prolactin in 50 per cent of patients.
B. Patients with a macroprolactinoma should start with a twice-daily dose of bromocriptine.
C. The starting dose of bromocriptine is 12.5 mg, given at night.
D. The usual starting dose of carbergoline is 0.25 mg twice weekly.

234. Haemoglobinopathies:
A. Sickle-cell disease is an autosomal recessive condition.
B. Sickle-cell disease during pregnancy is associated with higher risk of pulmonary embolism and renal infarction.
C. The alpha-thalassaemia gene is coded for by one gene on chromosome 16.
D. In beta-thalassaemia there are approximately 75 mutations responsible for the disorder.

235. The following are not common complications of cervical cancer:
A. Uraemia.
B. Pyometra.
C. Hydronephrosis.
D. Vesicocervical fistula.

236. Genetic disorders:
A. Beckwith–Weidemann syndrome is associated with exomphalos.
B. An affected male with cystic fibrosis is usually fertile.
C. Antenatal screening for cystic fibrosis is not possible.
D. Cystic hygroma is an autosomal recessive lesion.

237. Prostaglandin synthetase inhibitors:
A. Reduce menstrual blood loss by 20–50 per cent in 10 per cent of women.
B. Are more effective than tranexamic acid (TA) at reducing menstrual blood loss.
C. Inhibition of uterine prostaglandins reduces menstrual blood loss in less than 10 per cent of patients.
D. Side effects are more common with antifibrinolytics.

238. Hysteroscopic treatment for menorrhagia:
A. Is not an acceptable alternative to hysterectomy.
B. Offers a solution for menorrhagia as well as irreversible contraception.
C. Over 80 per cent of patients will have a lighter or no loss.
D. Patients exhibit a lower rate of postoperative infection than hysterectomy.
E. Cyclical pain improves after hysteroscopic treatment of dysfunctional uterine bleeding.
F. Radiofrequency ablation can destroy tissue up to a maximum depth of 7 mm.
G. Approximately 50 per cent of patients will eventually request further treatment after an endometrial ablative procedure.
H. Patients requiring hormone replacement therapy (HRT) after endometrial ablation should use a combined preparation.

239. Endometrial hyperplasia:
A. Will occur in 20 per cent of patients treated with unopposed oestrogen taken for 1 year.
B. Will develop into carcinoma in an average time of approximately 5 years.
C. 10 per cent of hyperplasia without atypia will progress to carcinoma.
D. If accompanied by atypia, 50 per cent will develop into carcinoma in 1 year.
E. The relative risk of developing endometrial carcinoma in women taking unopposed oestrogen is 6:1.
F. If repeat endometrial sampling shows normal or atrophic endometrium after 3–6 months of progesterone, no further treatment is required.

240. Androgens:

A. The majority of androgen production in women arises in the ovaries, under the influence of luteinizing hormone.

B. Sex hormone-binding globulin binds testosterone with high affinity, but not androstenedione.

C. Increased androgen production in hirsute women is commonly adrenal in origin.

D. Adrenal hyperandrogenaemia is found in about 15 per cent of patients with polycystic ovarian disease (PCOD).

241. Congenital adrenal hyperplasia (CAH):

A. Is most commonly caused by a deficiency of the 21-hydroxylase enzyme.

B. In adults is monitored by serum levels of 17-hydroxyprogesterone.

C. Is inherited in a recessive manner.

242. Prolactin:

A. Prolactin levels tend to be higher during the night.

B. Pregnancy is associated with a 10-fold increase in prolactin concentration.

243. Side effects of bromocriptine include:

A. Hypotension.

B. Nausea.

C. Miscarriage.

D. Congenital anomalies.

E. Multiple pregnancy.

244. The following statements are true about the preterm, breech fetus:

A. It should always be delivered by Caesarean section.

B. Cerebellar damage is a recognized complication of vaginal delivery.

C. Ultrasound is the best diagnostic tool in deciding which breech presentations may be permitted to deliver vaginally.

D. An experienced doctor should attend all vaginal deliveries.

E. Are best delivered by the vaginal route.

245. Congenital heart disease (CHD):

A. Is the commonest congenital malformation in children.

B. Is associated with an increased risk of aneuploidy.

C. Trisomy 13 (Patau's syndrome) is the most common aneuploidy associated with congenital heart disease.

D. Is more likely if there is increased nuchal translucency and a normal karyotype in the first trimester.

E. The four-chamber view of the fetal heart is a good screening test.

246. Kallman's syndrome is characterized by:

A. Precocious puberty.

B. Over-secretion of gonadotrophin-releasing hormone (GnRH).

C. Amenorrhoea.

D. Anosmia.

E. Genital hypertrophy.

247. **The following treatments are licensed for the prevention and treatment of osteoporosis:**
A. Etidronate (Didronel).
B. Alendronate (Fosamax).
C. Risedronate (Actonel).
D. Dietary calcium.
E. Raloxifene (Evista).

248. **The combined oral contraceptive pill (COCP) interacts with the following drugs:**
A. Barbiturates.
B. Rifampicin.
C. Aspirin.
D. Chloroquine.
E. Insulin.

249. **The following statements about molar pregnancy are true:**
A. The incidence of complete moles in the UK is 1:1200.
B. Partial moles are five times as common as complete moles.
C. Complete moles are diploid and androgenic in origin.
D. Partial moles are triploid conceptuses with two maternal haplotypes and one paternal set.
E. The incidence of molar pregnancy is dramatically decreased in women who conceive over the age of 50 years.

250. **Maternal steroid therapy:**
A. Decreases the incidence of intraventricular haemorrhage.
B. Is contraindicated in cases of prolonged preterm rupture of membranes.
C. Thyrotrophin-releasing hormone (TRH) is as effective as corticosteroids in inducing fetal lung maturity.
D. Reduces the incidence of respiratory distress syndrome in infants born preterm by 40–60 per cent.
E. For optimum results, steroids should be administered between 12 and 24 h prior to delivery.
F. Reduces the incidence of hypoxic ischaemic encephalopathy in the neonate.
G. Reduces the incidence of transient tachypnoea of the newborn.

251. **The intra-uterine contraceptive device (IUCD):**
A. If a patient is aged 40 years or over, there is no requirement to replace the device prior to the menopause.
B. Removal is not necessary in postmenopausal women.

252. **Ectopic pregnancy:**
A. If an intra-uterine sac is situated centrally, it is more likely to represent a pseudosac associated with ectopic pregnancy than an intra-uterine gestation.
B. The absence of a visible intra-uterine sac by transvaginal ultrasound, with a human chorionic gonadotrophin (hCG) level above 1000 IU/L is always a sign of an ectopic gestation.
C. In up to a quarter of patients with ectopic pregnancy, transvaginal ultrasound findings may be normal.

253. Neural tube defects:
A. Anencephaly and spina bifida account for more than 95 per cent of neural tube defects.
B. The incidence is higher in the USA and Canada than in the UK.
C. The recurrence risk if one sibling has been affected is 1:25.
D. The prognosis is poor if spina bifida is found in association with hydrocephalus.
E. The ultrasound finding of a banana-shaped cerebellum is a marker for spina bifida.
F. Preconceptual folic acid (500 micrograms per day) reduces the risk of recurrence.

254. The COCP and malignancy:
A. The COCP protects against ovarian cancer.
B. The COCP protects against breast cancer.
C. The COCP is associated with an increased risk of ovarian cancer.
D. The COCP is associated with a decreased risk of developing endometrial cancer.

255. Ovarian cancer:
A. Nulliparous women are at increased risk.
B. A personal history of breast cancer is associated with an increased risk.
C. Stage II disease is confined to the ovaries.
D. The 5-year survival rate for patients with stage IV disease is 70 per cent.
E. Tumours of low malignant potential are usually of the teratoma variety.

256. Preterm labour:
A. Is defined as regular uterine contractions and the presence of cervical dilatation occurring before 36 weeks' gestation.
B. A urinary tract infection is the aetiological factor in 90 per cent of cases.
C. Congenital anomalies are a risk factor for preterm labour.
D. Preterm labour affects 40 per cent of all pregnancies.
E. The main cause of perinatal morbidity is sepsis.
F. Tocolytics are not necessary after 30 weeks' gestation.

257. With regards to peritoneal healing:
A. After an intra-abdominal surgical procedure, it is complete within 5–8 days.
B. Non-closure of the peritoneum does not predispose patients to increased infectious complications.
C. Non-closure of the peritoneum decreases wound integrity.
D. Suturing of the peritoneum increases the incidence of adhesions postoperatively.
E. In the UK, the most common cause of intraperitoneal adhesion is a prior history of pelvic inflammatory disease.

258. Laparoscopic surgery:
A. Cutting diathermy uses high-current, low-voltage energy.
B. The pneumoperitoneum causes a widening of pulse pressure due to cardiac compression.
C. Peritoneal stretching commonly results in a tachycardia.
D. Increasing pain postoperatively represents perforation of the bowel until proven otherwise.
E. The aortic bifurcation occurs at the level of the iliac crest.

259. Early pregnancy:

A. If an embryo measures over 10 mm, the subsequent loss of viability is 0.5 per cent.
B. The finding of a well-defined regular endometrial line can effectively exclude incomplete miscarriage.
C. A missed miscarriage is defined as a fetal death before 20 weeks of gestation, without expulsion of the gestational sac.
D. A mean gestational sac diameter >20 mm is necessary before diagnosing missed miscarriage.
E. A gestational sac >25 mm with no fetal parts is termed a 'blighted ovum' or an 'anembryonic pregnancy'.

260. Thromboprophylaxis:

A. Patients with a history of a single episode of thromboembolism in pregnancy show a recurrence rate of 1–5 per cent.
B. Patients with a history of a single episode of thromboembolism in pregnancy should commence thromboprophylaxis as soon as pregnancy is diagnosed.
C. Antenatal low-dose heparin may cause thrombosis.
D. Warfarin used in the first trimester of pregnancy will produce central nervous system abnormalities in 46 per cent of fetuses.
E. Dextran 70 and hydration are recommended as the method of providing prophylaxis during labour and the early puerperium in mothers at low risk of thromboembolic disease.
F. In anti-thrombin III deficiency, the dose of heparin should be adjusted to maintain anti-factor 10a levels between 0.2–0.4 IU/mL.
G. Full anticoagulation is a clear contraindication to spinal or epidural anaesthesia.
H. In patients receiving heparin prophylaxis, the siting of an epidural or spinal block should be delayed for 24 h after the last low-dose heparin injection.
I. Low-dose heparin is associated with a 5–15 per cent increase in incidence of wound haematoma.

261. HIV-1 infection in pregnancy:

A. The human immunodeficiency virus is a retrovirus.
B. The CD4 lymphocyte is its main target.
C. AIDS occurs on average about 20 years after infection in adults.
D. In Europe the rate of vertical transmission is <5 per cent.
E. Caesarean section reduces the risk of infection from mother to infant by 20 per cent.

262. National Institute for Clinical Excellence (NICE) guidelines for induction of labour:

A. Dinoprostone and oxytocin are equally effective for the induction of labour after ruptured membranes, regardless of parity or cervical favourability.
B. Oxytocin may be started 4–6 h after vaginal prostaglandins.
C. The maximum recommended rate of oxytocin infusion is 20 milliunits/min (0.02 units/min).

263. In-vitro fertilization (IVF):
A. The success rate (take home baby rate) is 20 per cent.
B. The embryo is returned to the Fallopian tube.
C. Recovery of multiple oocytes allows cryopreservation of multiple embryos.
D. Bowel injury is a recognized complication of oocyte retrieval.

264. Anticholinergic drugs:
A. Produce competitive blockade of acetylcholine receptors.
B. Are specific for the bladder.
C. Should be stopped immediately if there is blurring of vision.
D. Should always be prescribed at the manufacturer's stated starting dose.
E. Cause antimuscarinic side effects.

265. Urodynamic investigation:
A. Detrusor instability is the commonest cause of incontinence and is defined as the presence of spontaneous detrusor contractions during the filling phase when the patient is attempting to inhibit micturition.
B. Genuine stress incontinence (GSI) is defined as the leakage of urine per urethra due to increased intra-abdominal pressure, in the absence of detrusor activity.
C. Has a relatively low sensitivity and specificity for detrusor instability.
D. A decreased maximum flow rate may indicate damage to the urethral sphincter.
E. Genuine stress incontinence can be diagnosed on an unlabelled urodynamic tracing.

266. Ectopic pregnancy:
A. The incidence has increased in the last decade.
B. Exposure to diethystilboestrol is a risk factor.
C. Most pregnancies occur in the fimbrial end of the tube.
D. At presentation, patients are usually mildly febrile.
E. Methotrexate is useful in the treatment of ectopic pregnancy due to its interference with RNA synthesis.

267. In the treatment of endometriosis:
A. Gestrinone is only administered twice weekly.
B. Gestrinone may increase libido.
C. Danazol may cause irreversible voice changes.
D. The benefits of luteinizing hormone-releasing hormone (LHRH) analogues are reduced by add-back oestrogen.

268. Hormone replacement therapy (HRT):
A. Reduces the risk of depressive symptoms.
B. Does not affect the incidence of Alzheimer's disease.
C. Does not reduce bone loss in the presence of established osteoporosis.
D. Retards the process leading to atheromatous plaque formation.
E. Lowers serum levels of high-density lipoprotein.
F. The minimum daily dose of oestradiol which prevents bone loss is 1 mg.
G. Is the first line of treatment in patients with established osteoporosis and fracture.
H. Tibolone does not provide effective relief from vasomotor symptoms.

269. Thrombophilic disorders:
A. Patients with anticardiolipin antibodies (ACA) are at increased risk of first- and second-trimester loss.
B. Patients with primary antiphospholipid syndrome (PAPS) are at increased risk of arterial, but not venous, thromboembolism.

270. Female sexual dysfunction:
A. May be caused by vaginismus.
B. Is successfully treated by sildenafil (Viagra).
C. Rarely has a physical cause.
D. Simple counselling and psychotherapy will help many couples.
E. Masters and Johnson working in the USA pioneered treatment for this disorder.

271. Premature rupture of membranes:
A. Is defined when the membranes rupture at the onset of preterm contractions.
B. Infection is occasionally implicated in its aetiology.
C. Infection decreases the production of prostaglandins in preterm ruptured membranes.
D. Is easy to diagnose conclusively.
E. Conservative management is the treatment of choice in all cases.
F. Culture of amniotic fluid is as useful to the paediatricians as to the obstetricians.
G. Vaginal flora is more abundant and homogenous in pregnancy.

272. Tocolytic therapy:
A. Magnesium sulphate is a recognized agent.
B. Oral tocolytic therapy has been proven to be of significant use in preterm labour.
C. Beta-sympathomimetic agonists function by reducing cyclic AMP in muscle cells and reducing intracellular calcium.
D. Free oral fluids should be encouraged.
E. Maternal blood glucose needs to be monitored.

273. Neonatal morbidity:
A. In the preterm baby, the commonest intracranial complication is subarachnoid haemorrhage.
B. Prematurity remains the commonest cause of neonatal death in the normally formed baby.
C. Preterm rupture of membranes needs to occur before 24 weeks' gestation to cause fetal lung hypoplasia.
D. Treatment of the mother with cortiosteroids antenatally reduces the risk of necrotizing enterocolitis.
E. Preterm delivery accounts for 35 per cent of perinatal deaths once congenital abnormality is excluded.
F. A subependymal haemorrhage (SEH) is defined as bleeding limited to the germinal matrix.
G. The end result of ischaemic brain injury is the formation of periventricular cysts (periventricular leukomalacia).
H. The incidence of retinopathy of prematurity is approximately 13 per cent at 25 weeks.

274. Pulmonary physiology:
A. A lecithin/sphingomyelin (L/S) ratio of 0.5 indicates a low risk of respiratory distress syndrome.
B. Lecithin is produced by type I pneumocytes in the lungs.
C. The lecithin/sphingomyelin ratio is a reliable test of lung maturity.
D. At 32–34 weeks' gestation the respiratory epithelial cells start to differentiate into type I and type II pneumocytes.
E. Type 1 pneumocytes in the fetus are concerned with gas exchange.
F. Bronchopulmonary dysplasia (BPD) is defined as oxygen dependency at 36 weeks' postmenstrual age in babies who survive respiratory distress syndrome.
G. Approximately 25 per cent of babies born below 25 weeks develop chronic lung disease (CLD).

275. Cervical incompetence:
A. Is characterized by painful cervical dilatation in the second trimester.
B. May be caused by diethylstilboestrol.
C. LLETZ (large loop excision of the transformation zone) is commonly associated.
D. May be treated with intravenous ritodrine.

276. The preterm neonate:
A. Suffers thermal stress because of its low surface area-to-mass ratio.
B. Surfactant production increases as its temperature drops.
C. Lower core temperature is associated with a decreased oxygen and glucose consumption.

277. Endometrial carcinoma:
A. The histological grade of tumour is one of the most important prognostic factors.
B. 50 percent of patients with clinical stage 1 disease have positive peritoneal cytology.
C. The risk of recurrent disease is increased three-fold with positive peritoneal cytology.
D. Patients with oestrogen/progesterone receptor positive tumours frequently have poorly differentiated tumours with marked invasiveness.
E. Approximately 25 per cent of tumours exhibit DNA aneuploidy.

278. Ca125 (normal range <35 U/mL):
A. May be elevated with menstruation.
B. Is raised in 50 per cent of stage I ovarian cancers.
C. Is elevated in pelvic inflammatory disease (PID).
D. May be raised by urinary tract infection.
E. Is elevated in patients with pancreatic cancer.

279. Amniocentesis:
A. There is a procedure-related miscarriage rate of approximately 0.1 per cent.
B. FISH (fluorescence in-situ hybridization) may be used to exclude the more common aneuploidies.
C. The cell culture will fail in approximately 5 per cent of samples.

280. The following are features of babies born with trisomy 18 (Edward's syndrome):
A. Rocker bottom feet.
B. Intra-uterine growth retardation.
C. Polydactyly.
D. A strawberry-shaped head on prenatal ultrasound.

281. Neurofibromatosis type I:
A. Is an autosomal dominant disorder.
B. May be associated with renal artery stenosis and phaeochromocytoma.
C. Has a very high association with malignancy.

282. Pre-implantation genetic diagnosis:
A. The technique involves the removal of one or two blastomeres from the embryo on day 3 of development.
B. Is not possible for Duchenne's muscular dystrophy.
C. Is regulated by the HFEA (Human Fertilisation and Embryology Authority), from whom a license must be obtained on a case-by-case basis.
D. May be used to identify single-gene defects.
E. Less than 1 per cent of newborns have a single minor malformation.

283. Placental abruption
A. The risk of recurrence is 8.3–16.7 per cent.
B. The commonest reason is blunt trauma to the abdomen.
C. Causes are usually obvious clinically.
D. Many patients with placental abruption are hypertensive at presentation.
E. Nearly 50 per cent of patients are in established labour.
F. Approximately 10 per cent of patients are in established labour.

284. Acute fatty liver and pregnancy:
A. The major risk of acute fatty liver of pregnancy is maternal death.
B. The major risk of acute fatty liver of pregnancy is fetal death in up to 40 per cent of cases.
C. Liver enzymes (AST: aspartate transaminase and ALT: alanine transaminase) are usually markedly elevated.

285. Contraindications to the progesterone pill:
A. Patients with porphyria.
B. Patients suffering from migraine.
C. A history of severe arterial disease.

Answers

1.

A. True.

B. True.

C. True.

D. True.

E. True.

2.

A. **True.** Antihistamines such as chlorpheniramine and terfenadine are thought to be safe during pregnancy.

B. **True.** In the CLASP study (1995) there was no significant problem. However, it may lead to haemorrhage due to impaired platelet function.

C. **False.** Vitamin A is found in high concentrations in the liver and cod liver oil capsules; these should be avoided in early pregnancy.

D. **False.**

E. **False.** Live vaccines, such as BCG, MMR, oral polio, oral typhoid and yellow fever should be avoided if possible.

F. **False.**

Timing of exposure to 'teratogen'

Pre-embryonic phase (days 0–14 after conception): all or nothing effect.

Embryonic phase (weeks 3–8): the time of the greatest theoretical risk of congenital malformation.

Fetal phase (weeks 9 to birth): fetal growth and development can be impaired by drugs, but fetal malformation unlikely.

3.

A. **True.** The vacuum extractor should not be used in situations where dystocia is thought to be due to cephalopelvic disproportion, or where fetal position cannot be confidently determined. In addition, it should not be used to deliver a premature fetus, since the incidence of serious fetal injury is probably increased in these cases.

B. **False.** It describes failure of the vertex to descend with the sagittal suture in the midplane between front and back of the pelvis.

C. **True.** The anterior fontanelle is felt to be low in the pelvis as opposed to an anterior position with a well-flexed head.

D. **True.** Other signs include excessive back pain and the possibility of poor progress in labour because of the larger occipitofrontal diameter of 11 cm associated with the deflexed head.

4.
A. **True.**
B. **False.** First-degree prolapse is to the level of the ischial spine.
C. **False.**
D. **False.** Cystocoele presents thus. Rectocele involves protrusion of the posterior vaginal wall.
E. **False.** Vault prolapse involves descent of the cuff of vaginal tissue left after hysterectomy.
F. **True.** The levator ani muscle, which forms this support, comprises ischiococcygeus, iliococcygeus and pubococcygeus.
G. **False.** Procidentia refers to the descent of the cervix and the uterus through the introitus.
H. **True.** Prolapse of the upper two-thirds is termed a cystocele.
I. **True.** In contrast to a rectocele which describes prolapse of the posterior vaginal wall.
J. **True.** Vaginal hysterectomy is also a useful treatment option where an enterocele is present as the uterosacral ligaments may be used to repair the hernial sac.
K. **False.** Cystourethrocele is most common. An urethrocele occurring alone is unusual.
L. **True.** Estimating the appropriate size when fitting a ring pessary for the first time is facilitated by measuring this distance at vaginal examination and choosing a ring of equal diameter.
M. **True.** It may be considered in patients with severe prolapse who wish to have more children. Delivery of these children should be by Caesarean section.
N. **True.** The peritoneum forms a hernial sac with the said contents.

5.
A. **True.** The anti-endometriosis drug, danazol, is a testosterone derivative that has weak androgenic activity and may result in cliteromegaly and labial fusion with female fetal exposure. Apparently this agent has no adverse effects in male fetuses exposed *in utero*.
B. **True.** The two most common features are nasal hypoplasia and stippling of epiphyses. This anticoagulant may also result in adverse fetal effects such as intracerebral haemorrhage, microcephaly, cataracts, blindness and mental retardation when utilized during the second or third trimester of pregnancy.
C. **True.** Most antineoplastics have been reported to be teratogenic in humans. In particular, folate antagonists (e.g. aminopterin and methotrexate) are very well known human teratogens.
D. **True.** Tetracyclines are the only antibacterial agents known to have teratogenic effects. Fortunately, the discoloration of the deciduous teeth is purely cosmetic and does not affect permanent teeth.
E. **True.** Use of this agent during early gestation is reportedly associated with an increased risk of cardiovascular anomalies in exposed offspring.

6.

A. **False.** Recent evidence suggests that magnesium sulphate is the treatment of choice in patients with actual seizure activity.

B. **False.**

C. **False.**

D. **False.**

E. **True.**

Treatment of eclampsia

Magnesium sulphate is the treatment of choice in patients with actual seizures (eclampsia). The recently published MAGPIE trial (Lancet 2002) confirms that magnesium sulphate is also safe to use in pre-eclampsia and will prevent 50 per cent of seizures.

Beta-blockers may cause intra-uterine growth restriction, neonatal hypoglycaemia, and bradycardia; the risk is greater in severe hypertension.

7.

A. **False.** Growth (anagen), hairfall (catogen) and resting (telogen) take up to 3 years.

B. **False.** 1 cm.

C. **False.** Androgens increase sebum production, leading to comedones and acne, and provoke terminal hair growth – except on the scalp, where hair loss can occur in a male pattern.

D. **True.** Excess hair is not always 'male pattern'.

E. **False.** These pigmented velvety patches are found in the skin flexures and neck, and suggest polycystic ovarian syndrome (PCOS) and insulin resistance.

F. **True.**

G. **False.** These conditions must be distinguished, as they do not respond to anti-androgens.

8.

A. **False.** It is probably due to maternal auto-antibodies.

B. **False.** NLE is rare (1:20 000 live births).

C. **False.** The typical skin lesions include erythematous, scaling annular or elliptical plaques occurring on the face or scalp.

Neonatal lupus erythematosus

A spectrum of neonatal autoimmune sequelae can result from maternal systemic lupus erythematosus (SLE) due to transplacental neonatal passage of pathogenic auto-antibodies or possibly of immune complexes. This spectrum ranges from neonatal discoid lupus which is transient and benign, to a lupus systemic disorder characterized by hepatosplenomegaly, anaemia, thrombocytopenia, generalized skin lesions and congenital complete heart block. Neonatal death from the systemic syndrome is usual, but not invariable.

9.

A. **False.** Fetal fibronectin is a component of the extracellular matrix of the cervix. If fibronectin is found in cervical samples, then onset of labour is more likely. It has a positive predictive value for preterm delivery in high-risk patients of 46 per cent. The inclusion of this test in assessment of preterm labour is as yet controversial due to its low sensitivity.

B. **False.** Evidence is conflicting. The 1995 Collaborative Home Uterine Monitoring Study failed to find significant differences between monitoring and sham monitoring.

C. **False.** Diagnosis of spontaneous rupture of the membranes by nitrazene test has 15 per cent false-positive rate.

10.

A. **False.** Facultative anaerobic. Important pathogenic species for man include Group A (*Streptococcus pyogenes*), Group B (*Streptococcus agalactiae*) and Group D (enterococci).

B. **False.**

C. **True.**

D. **True.** May be arranged in pairs or chains.

E. **False.** Potassium hydroxide demonstrates typical mycelial forms and pseudohyphae in 80 per cent of patients with symptomatic candida infection. Identification of GBS is based on the presence of polysaccharide group specific antigen (serologic testing). Group B can be further subdivided into types – Ia, Ib, Ic, II, III.

F. **True.** Vaginal or cervical contamination and colonization occur from a gastro-intestinal tract source. The frequency of GBS isolation increases as one proceeds from the cervix to the introitus, and GBS can be recovered twice as frequently from rectal cultures as from vaginal cultures.

Group B haemolytic *Streptococcus* (GBS)

Gram +ve cocci

Facultative anaerobes

Non-motile

Arranged in chains

11.

A. **True.** Hypertension and advanced parity are associated with an increased risk of abruption.

B. **True.** This is thought to be due to its hypertensive effect.

C. **True.** The rate of abruption is five times that of an uncomplicated pregnancy.

D. **True.** It is a risk factor for placental abruption, but protective against the development of pre-eclampsia. However, if pre-eclampsia occurs it tends to be more severe.

E. **False.** Trauma, notably in the form of road traffic accidents, may cause placental abruption and many other factors are implicated.

F. **True.** The risk of abruption is increased where the site of placenta attachment covers a fibroid.

G. **False.** It occurs more frequently in older women, but this increase has been attributed to parity, and is independent of age.

12.
A. **True.** Genetic factors play a more important role in the first half of pregnancy.
B. **True.** The average difference is 150–200 g.
C. **False.** Maternal heart rate and blood pressure increase.
D. **True.**
E. **False.** This indicates high resistance within the uterine artery, possibly due to failure of trophoblastic invasion.
F. **False.** Birthweight tends to rise; possibly as maternal weight increases between the first and second pregnancies.

13.
A. **True.** But the incidence is greater with monochorionicity.
B. **True.** Different sex fetuses are always dichorionic and dizygous.
C. **False.** The figure is true for the monochorionic twin pregnancy, while the incidence in the dichorionic is 1.8 per cent.

Twins with one fetal death

If death occurs in the first or early second trimester there may be no adverse consequences on the survivor.

If fetal loss occurs in the late second or third trimester it commonly precipitates labour, and 90 per cent will deliver within 3 weeks.

The prognosis for the surviving twin is influenced by its gestation, but many are irreversibly damaged by the sudden haemodynamic changes arising from the death of its partner or by circulating toxins produced by the dead twin.

In monochorionic twins there are risks of death and cerebral damage.

14.
A. **True.**
B. **False.** 0.6 and 0.8 kg/cm^2.
C. **False.** 3 cm anterior to the posterior fontanelle.
D. **True.** Increasing the vacuum in two steps is not necessary: the pressure may be set to the desired maximum immediately. Two minutes is enough time to allow a good chignon to develop (Vacca, 1992).

> **Vacuum extractor**
>
> **Advantages:**
>
> Easy application, autorotation of the malpositioned fetal head, safety to both mother and fetus.
>
> **Disadvantages:**
>
> *Maternal*
>
> Vaginal and cervical laceration.
>
> *Fetal*
>
> The formation of the chignon, the oedematous artificial caput formed beneath the vaccum cup.
>
> Fetal scalp laceration and abrasions.
>
> Cephalhaematomas are more common, but apart from causing neonatal jaundice are rarely of clinical significance.

15.

A. **True.** Other sites commonly involved are the ligaments (uterosacral, round and broad) and Fallopian tubes as well as pelvic peritoneum.

B. **True.** This is usually achieved by biopsy at the time of laparoscopy.

C. **False.** Disease severity correlates very poorly with pain experienced. Some patients with endometriosis visible at laparoscopy are asymptomatic, except for having problems with fertility.

D. **False.**

E. **False.**

F. **False.**

G. **False.**

H. **False.** Mobile retroversion is a normal finding in approximately 20 per cent of women. Fixed retroversion is usually secondary to underlying disease, e.g. endometriosis.

> **Risk factors for endometriosis:**
>
> *Increased risk*
>
> Japanese race, family history, oestrogen status, age 30–44 years, increased menstrual flow and decreased cycle length, environmental factors, alcohol, increased peripheral body fat.
>
> *Decreased risk*
>
> Current and recent oral contraceptive users, current IUCD users, possibly smokers.

16.

A. **True.** This agent is no longer commercially available for use as a sedative, but is used in the therapy for tuberculosis.

B. **True.** Between days 27 and 42 post conception.

C. **False.** Absence of the long bones.

D. **True.**

Terminology of limb defects

- Acromelia: shortening predominantly of distal segments.
- Rhizomelia: shortening predominantly in proximal long bones.
- Mesomelia: shortening predominantly in the intermediate long bone.
- Amelia: absence of a limb.
- Hemimelia: absence or hypoplasia of longitudinal segments.
- Phocomelia: absence or hypoplasia of long bones with hands or feet attached to trunk.
- Kyphosis: dorsally convex curvature of spine.
- Lordosis: dorsally concave curvature of the spine.
- Scoliosis: lateral curvature of the spine.

17.

A. **False.** Insulin antagonizes the action of cortisol on lecithin synthesis by cultured fetal lung cells.

B. **True.** Several studies have suggested that fetal hyperinsulinaemia may be associated with delayed appearance of PG and an increased incidence of respiratory distress syndrome.

C. **True.** The action of lecithin is dependent on phosphatidyl inositol (secreted in the second trimester) and phosphatidyl glycerol (secreted mainly in the last 5 weeks of pregnancy). The relative deficiency of phosphatidyl glycerol in diabetic pregnancies may lead to respiratory distress syndrome, despite a 'mature' lecithin:sphingomyelin ratio.

Surfactant

Lung alveoli are lined by a group of phospholipids known collectively as surfactant. The predominant phospholipid (80 per cent) is dipalmitoylphosphatidyl choline (lecithin). There is a surge of lecithin production at 35–36 weeks of fetal life. The surge can be promoted by cortisol, growth retardation and prolonged rupture of membranes, and is delayed in diabetes. Others phospholipids are sphingomyelin, phosphatidylglycerol and phosphatidylinositol. Sphingomyelin production reaches a peak at about 32 weeks and diminishes after 35 weeks. The lecithin:sphingomyelin ratio provides a measure of lung maturity.

18.

A. **True.** Hysterectomy is the safest method of treatment. If uterine function must be preserved, it is possible to leave the placenta *in situ*. Complete autolysis may occur, or treatment with methotrexate has been described.

B. **True.** It is probably due to a deficiency of decidua in the lower uterine segment.

C. **True.** ·

> ### Placenta accreta
>
> • Pathological adherence due to the paucity of underlying decidua.
>
> *Types of placenta accreta:*
>
> • Placenta increta: the placenta invades the uterine wall.
>
> • Placenta percreta: the invasion reaches the uterine serosa and may even lead to rupture of the uterus.

19.

A. **True.** And/or fasting glucose is >7.8 mmol/L.

B. **False.** Insulin should be administered as an intravenous infusion combined with intravenous glucose.

C. **True.** 10 per cent glucose should be used at a fixed rate of 100 mL every hour, and adjusted to maintain blood glucose concentration at 4–6 mmol/L.

D. **True.** This, in association with glycosuria, predisposes the patient to monilial vaginitis and vulvitis.

E. **True.**

F. **False.** Increased ×3. The commonest congenital malformations are cardiovascular system, skeletal and central nervous system.

20.

A. **True.** Endometrial carcinomas in patients taking unopposed oestrogens tend to be well differentiated.

B. **False.**

C. **True.** These carcinomas regress more readily with progestogen therapy.

D. **False.** They carry a good prognosis.

E. **False.** Recurrence is uncommon.

21.

A. **False.** Hypertension is the one of the commonest complications of pregnancy. It is associated with fetal and maternal mortality and morbidity. 5–15 per cent of cases are associated with proteinuria, in which case fetal and maternal risks are increased. 80 per cent of normal pregnant women exhibit oedema. Even when associated with hypertension and proteinuria, it is not of prognostic significance.

B. **False.** The point of disappearance of the Korotkoff sounds (point V) in patients who are not pregnant matches the true DBP as measured by intra-arterial catheter. In pregnancy, the Korotkoff sounds may persist to zero due to the marked peripheral vasodilatation. Thus, diastolic pressure is taken to be muffling of the sounds (point IV).

C. **False.** Hypertension in pregnancy is subclassified as essential, pregnancy-induced, pregnancy-induced with proteinuria, essential, transient, and that associated with chronic renal disease.

D. **True.** Transient hypertension is a diagnosis of exclusion. The true definition is third-trimester elevation of blood pressure without evidence of pre-eclampsia in a patient who has been proven to be normotensive when not pregnant. Often, transient hypertension is a diagnosis made in retrospect.

E. **False.** Transient hypertension is only one part of pregnancy-induced hypertension, which includes patients with proteinuria.

F. **False.** The pregnancy is at risk for intra-uterine growth restriction, abruption, and stillbirth because of poor placental vascular development and ongoing elevations of blood pressure. Maternal complications include superimposed pre-eclampsia and the associated consequences. Many clinicians hold that superimposed pre-eclampsia is of greater clinical significance than simple pre-eclampsia.

G. **True.** Patients with chronic hypertension should have their blood pressure under control when they conceive. They should continue antihypertensive drugs when they are pregnant, even when blood pressure drops to normal range in the second trimester. The exceptions are drugs associated with congenital anomalies or adverse fetal outcomes – such as angiotensin-converting enzyme (ACE) inhibitors. In this case, another medication should be substituted.

22.

A. **False.** Epithelial ovarian carcinoma staging is used in both cases.

B. **True.** This is particularly so in pregnancy. Pain and bleeding result.

C. **False.** The definition is correct except the ovarian tumour is benign (fibroma).

D. **True.** Other primary tumours metastasizing to ovary include breast, female genital tract, leukaemia and lymphoma.

E. **False.** The primary sites involved also include colon, breast and biliary tract. The diagnosis hinges on mucin-containing signet ring cells and a sarcoma-like stromal hyperplasia.

Ovarian cancer

The commonest sites for the primary carcinoma metastasizing to the ovary are the stomach, colon, breast, uterus, Fallopian tube and the opposite ovary. The breast is the most frequent site.

Krukenberg tumours

These account for 30–40 per cent of metastic cancer. The lesion consists of clumps and cords of epithelial cells in a proliferating stroma. They are characterized by 'signet ring' cells – epithelial cells bloated with mucin and having an eccentric nucleus. The primary growth is always in mucin-secreting tissue, usually the stomach or colon, but sometimes the gallbladder or breast.

Meigs' syndrome

- Fibroma is one of the few benign tumours of the ovary which causes ascites in 20 per cent of cases.
- Associated hydrothorax is common.

23.

A. **False.** The contraceptive effect is more dependent upon endometrial and cervical mucus effects, since gonadotrophins are not consistently suppressed. Approximately 40 per cent of patients will ovulate normally.

B. **True.** High-dose progestogens suppress pituitary gonadotrophins, and therefore ovulation ceases.

C. **False.** Progesterone-only methods that do not inhibit ovulation are associated with functional ovarian cysts.

24.

A. **True.** There is no evidence to suggest it is a human teratogen, but there may be adverse neonatal effects with high doses of the drug administered to the mother near the time of delivery. It is rarely utilized because of the risk of maternal aplastic anaemia and 'grey-baby syndrome' in the newborn.

B. **True.** The sulpha part leads to kernicterus due to bilirubin displacement; trimethoprim is a weak folate antagonist, but has not been found to be associated with an increased risk of congenital anomalies.

C. **False.** The benefit of treatment of malaria infection far outweighs the risks. Chloroquine is preferred as prophylaxis.

D. **False.** All of the penicillins are apparently safe for use during pregnancy in patients not allergic to these drugs.

E. **True.** Associated with transient haemolytic anaemia.

F. **False.**

G. **True.** Associated with irreversible arthropathy.

> **Antibiotics with potentially adverse effects include:**
> - Tetracyclines: yellow-brown discoloration of the deciduous teeth.
> - Aminoglycosides: ototoxicity (VIII cranial nerve damage).
> - Sulphonamides: hyperbilirubinaemia, transient.
> - Nitrofurantoin: haemolytic anaemia, transient.
> - Fluoroquinolones: irreversible arthropathy.
> - MTT-containing cephalosporins: testicular hypoplasia.
>
> *Augmentation*
>
> The British National Formulary states that all cephalosporins are safe in pregnancy. MTT stands for n-methyl tetrathiazole, a molecular side chain. It is found in cefoperazole, cefamandole and moxalactam. There is no evidence that the addition of the side chain causes damage to the unborn fetus as there have been no human studies. In animal studies male rats may develop testicular hypoplasia and be infertile.

25.
A. **True.**   As are the limb buds.
B. **False.**   This occurs at 7 weeks.
C. **True.**   At this stage it is also possible to see the knees, elbows, crossed legs, stomach and choroid plexus. At 10 weeks, the heart chambers, bladder and kidneys are visible.
D. **True.**   As in the non-pregnant state, but one ovary is usually seen to contain one larger cystic structure, the corpus luteal cyst.
E. **False.**   A small amount of free fluid may be seen within the pouch of Douglas in normal pregnancy.

26.
A. **True.**   Uterine anomalies and fetal anomalies predispose to breech presentation.
B. **True.**
C. **True.**
D. **True.**

27.
A. **True.**   An echogenic focus is a moving echogenic focus within one or both cardiac ventricles, which has no obvious anatomically associated structure. It may represent papillary microcalcification.
B. **True.**   In such instances, it is important to exclude structural heart disease.

28.

A. **False.** Compensatory changes occur in the circulation in an attempt to maintain adequate tissue oxygenation. Plasma volume and cardiac output rise, peripheral resistance falls, and the velocity of blood flow increases. In severe anaemia, compensation by these means is not adequate.

B. **True.** And the same survival time as in the non-pregnant state.

C. **False.** A haemoglobin concentration of <10 g/dL and a haematocrit of <35 per cent are the criteria for diagnosing pregnancy anaemia.

D. **True.** It is also thought to increase the risk of thromboembolism; in mothers with cardiac or respiratory disease, it predisposes to decompensation.

E. **True.** Each fetus and placenta requires about 500 mg of iron, and a similar amount is needed for the red cell increment. Average postpartum blood loss and lactation for 6 months each account for about 180 mg.

F. **False.** The therapeutic optimal daily intake of elemental iron is 100 mg.

G. **False.** Ferrous salts are much better absorbed: ferrous sulphate and ferrous fumarate. Absorption may be increased by adding ascorbic acid (vitamin C).

H. **False.** Iron is absorbed in the stomach and first part of the duodenum. Modified-release preparations carry the iron past the duodenum, reducing both absorption and side effects.

29.

A. **True.** Which is 1000 times greater than after a normal pregnancy.

B. **True.**

C. **False.** These tumours have the potential of developing metastatic disease, and the sonographic appearance is of small, localized, fluid-filled cysts, similar to an invasive mole within the uterus.

Factors increasing the risk of needing chemotherapy include (*Dewhurst's Textbook of Obstetrics and Gynaecology for Postgraduates*, 6th edn):

- Beta-hCG level >100 000 IU/L pre evacuation.
- Uterine size greater than gestational age.
- Theca lutein cysts >6 cm diameter.
- Maternal age greater than 40 years.
- Previous molar pregnancy.
- Hyperthyroidism.
- Trophoblastic emboli.
- Disseminated intravascular coagulation.
- Toxaemia.

D. **True.** Sonographically, choriocarcinoma can be discovered within the pelvis or other distant organs. It is composed of necrotic tissue and haemorrhage which produce a sonographic picture of a semi-solid echogenic mass.

Trophoblastic disease

- Invasive hydatidiform mole may be complete or partial. This is common, as molar trophoblast invades the myometrium in most cases. A pathological diagnosis can only be made if an adequate sample of myometrium is available within the curettings or at time of hysterectomy.

- Choriocarcinoma is a tumour involving both cyto-trophoblast and syncytio-trophoblast cells. At microscopy, scattered tumour cells are visualized within a haemorrhagic, necrotic mass. Interpretation can be difficult as tumour cells may be few in number. Intravascular dissemination can be widespread including to lung and brain.

- Placental site trophoblastic tumours are rare and contain mostly cytotrophoblastic cells. They do not metastasize as widely as choriocarcinoma, but tend to invade locally. Optimal management is as yet uncertain, but may involve hysterectomy and/or chemotherapy. (Trophoblastic Tumour Screening and Treatment Centre, Charing Cross Hospital; www.hmole-chorio.org.uk)

30.
A. **True.** All major structures in the body will be formed in the first 12 weeks. Thus, drug treatment before this time may cause teratogenic effects.
B. **True.** Use lignocaine or bupivacaine instead as local anaesthesia.
C. **True.** In addition, renal function impairment and persistent pulmonary hypertension in the newborn.
D. **True.** Podophyllum is an antimitotic agent.
E. **True.**
F. **True.** In addition they may lead to neonatal irritability and muscle spasms.

Anaesthesia during pregnancy

The effect mainly during the third trimester:

- General: depress neonatal respiration.

- Local: with large doses, neonatal respiratory depression, hypotonia, and bradycardia after paracervical or epidural block; neonatal methaemoglobinaemia with prilocaine and procaine.

31.
A. **False.** Three randomized controlled trials have shown no effect of early version on incidence of breech birth, Caesarean section rates, or postnatal outcome.
B. **False.** The correct figure is 50 per cent.
C. **True.** Both fetal mortality and morbidity are associated with external cephalic version.
D. **True.** These complications occur in approximately 3 out of every 1000 versions.

32.
A. **True.** Reflecting our poor understanding of the pathophysiology.
B. **False.** Anterior colporrhaphy is the operation of choice for anterior vaginal wall prolapse, but not GSI.
C. **False.** 8 per cent.
D. **True.**
E. **True.** Urethro-vaginal fistula in 0.3 per cent, long-term voiding difficulty in 12 per cent, de-novo detrusor instability in 11 per cent. However, the cure rate is approaching 90 per cent.
F. **False.** The disadvantage of this operation is that it is unable to correct a cystocele.

33.
A. **True.** In non-pregnant subjects the minimum daily requirement for folate is about 50 micrograms. Increased demands in pregnancy are associated with falling blood levels and morphological changes in the red and white blood cells by the end of pregnancy or postpartum.
B. **False.** Before the introduction of folic acid supplementation in the UK, the incidence of megaloblastic anaemia in pregnancy was between 0.5 and 3.0 per cent.
C. **True.** Anticonvulsant drugs may inhibit the utilization of folic acid in the marrow. Thus, the requirement for folic acid is increased. Gluten sensitivity is the usual cause in non-tropical countries.
D. **True.** Some patients are very ill with obvious anaemia and dyspnoea. The tongue is usually painful and shows some papillary flattening, or it may be 'mapped' with dark red patches. Aphthous ulceration of the tongue and mouth is common. Liver and spleen enlargement may not be easy to detect in late pregnancy. There may be protracted vomiting, and anorexia is prominent in most patients.
E. **False.** Chronic haemolytic anaemias such as sickle-cell disease or beta-thalassaemia are likely to lead to severe folate depletion.
F. **False.** The fetus obtains enough folic acid of its own, regardless of the severity of maternal deficiency.
G. **False.** Folic acid deprivation leads after several weeks to reduced serum folate, soon followed by hypersegmentation of the neutrophils. Later, the blood film will show anisocytosis and macrocytosis.

Folic acid

A normal Western diet contains 500–700 micrograms folic acid per day, of which between 10 and 100 per cent may be lost in cooking. Requirements increase during pregnancy (400–800 micrograms/day) and can be met by supplements of 200–300 micrograms/day. Folic acid absorbed from the diet is reduced in the tissues to the active form, tetrahydrofolic acid. Folate is actively transported by the placenta to the fetus, and the maternal plasma folate level falls by almost half during pregnancy (from 6 micrograms/L to 3.5 micrograms/L).

34.

A. **False.** Urethral pressures are not an essential part of urodynamic investigation.

B. **True.** There is considerable overlap between normal and GSI individuals. If it is very low, it suggests that a colposuspension may fail and that a sling should be performed, but this hypothesis has yet to be properly tested.

C. **True.** Dipstick urine testing correlates well with UTI. If positive, urodynamics should be postponed.

D. **True.** Urodynamics does cause iatrogenic infection. It may be as much as 10 per cent but the reported range is wide (2–10 per cent).

E. **False.** In the absence of a rise in detrusor pressure

35.

A. **False.** Recurrent miscarriage is defined as the loss of three or more consecutive pregnancies.

B. **False.** Between 12 per cent and 15 per cent of clinically recognized pregnancies miscarry. Therefore, the expected chance of three consecutive pregnancy losses is 0.3 per cent. However, 1 per cent of couples suffer from recurrent miscarriage.

C. **False.** The traditionally held beliefs that diabetes mellitus and thyroid dysfunction are associated with recurrent miscarriage are not supported by the available data. Untreated diabetes mellitus and thyroid disease are implicated.

D. **False.** 5 per cent of women with a history of recurrent miscarriage, 4 per cent amongst a control group, and 20 per cent in women with a history of second trimester miscarriage.

E. **True.**

F. **True.** Varying causes are identified including genetic causes, endocrine problems and autoimmune disease.

Protocol for the investigation of women with a history of recurrent miscarriage (all patients)

RCOG Guidelines, 1998.

Investigation	Problem detected by Investigation	Women with problem (%)
Karyotyping (both partners)	Chromosome abnormality	3–5
Karotyping of fetal products	Chromosome abnormality	
Pelvic ultrasound	Polycystic ovarian disease (PCOD)	56
Lupus anticoagulant Anticardiolipin antibody	Antiphosphilipid antibodies	15

36.
A. **False.** The frequency of diagnosis decreases during pregnancy. However, this does not mean that ulcers cannot occur *de novo*.
B. **True.** This is due to folic acid deficiency, which may also cause megaloblastic anaemia.
C. **False.** The risk of exacerbation is not necessarily increased by pregnancy, although active disease in early pregnancy is more likely to be followed by a flare in later pregnancy or in the postnatal period. Relapses of ulcerative colitis are not ameliorated by termination of pregnancy.

37.
A. **False.** This triad occurs in the third trimester.
B. **False.** Proteinuria of more than 5 g in 24 h is the criterion.
C. **True.** Other risk factors for pre-eclampsia include diabetes, multiple gestations and chronic hypertension.
D. **True.** However, in the patient with recurrent pre-eclampsia, underlying maternal disease may be at fault and may have implications for later life.
E. **True.** Fibronectin is a glycoprotein involved in platelet activation, the coagulation cascade and intercellular adhesion. As fibronectin is a component of collagen, the elevated plasma levels probably reflect the endothelial damage, which is thought to be the primary pathology underlying pre-eclampsia.
F. **False.** It usually precedes the development of proteinuria, and is a simple investigation.

38.
A. **False.** Clam iliocystoplasty is currently the operation of choice for intractable detrusor instability. It is not indicated for idiopathic urgency or for urgency of neuropathic origin.
B. **True.**
C. **False.** Genuine stress incontinence constitutes 75–80 per cent of these cases.
D. **True.** These patients often show bladder capacity of less than 300 mL.
E. **True.**

39.
A. **False.**
B. **False.**
C. **False.** Oestrogens by themselves aggravate endometriosis, but the combined oral contraceptive pill causes shrinkage of normal and ectopic endometrium.

40.

A. **False.** The clinical use of the drug has been limited by its dose-related androgenic side effects.

B. **False.** They are dose-related.

C. **False.** Ovarian suppression and amenorrhoea, with the associated problems of the hypoestrogenic state including hot flushes, vaginal dryness and bone mineral loss, mean that GnRH analogues are clearly not the medical therapy of choice for all women with menorrhagia. However, they may have a place for short-term treatment.

D. **True.** Hypo-oestrogenic symptoms may be overcome by the simultaneous prescription of synthetic progestogens or combined hormone replacement therapy.

E. **False.** Agents such as danazol or GnRH analogues result in marked reductions in blood loss or amenorrhoea. However, these medications are not appropriate as first-line treatments or for long-term administration for menorrhagia. Their main use in current clinical settings is in preparation for hysteroscopic treatment of menorrhagia.

Medical treatments for menorrhagia include:

- Prostaglandin synthetase inhibitors (e.g. mefenamic acid).
- Antifibrinolytic agents (e.g. tranexamic acid).
  - Hormonal treatments:
  - combined contraceptive pill;
  - synthetic progestogens;
  - levonorgestrel intra-uterine system;
  - danazol;
  - gonadotrophin-releasing hormone analogues.

41.

A. **True.** Following a partial mole, approximately 0.5 per cent will require treatment. Both these conditions need to be monitored by serial hCG estimations to confirm that they have regressed and have gone into complete remission.

B. **True.** Because it may stimulate molar tissue to regrow as choriocarcinoma.

C. **False.** Once hCG has returned to normal, the COCP is not contraindicated.

D. **True.** Given as an 8-day course with methotrexate given on days 1, 3, 5 and 7, and folinic acid rescue on days 2, 4, 6 and 8 with these courses repeated on a 2-week cycle.

E. **True.** Side effects include alopecia and, rarely, myelosuppression.

42.

A. **False.** However, some will be infertile and some will undergo a premature menopause.

B. **True.** The younger the patient, the less chance of permanent amenorrhoea.

43.

A. **False.** Incidental thrombocytopenia of pregnancy is a common occurrence (5 per cent). The platelet count is usually $>80 \times 10^9$/L.

B. **True.** And is also associated with transverse myelitis, autoimmune haemolytic anaemia and chorea gravidarum.

C. **False.** However, the risk of haemorrhage increases due to issues related to pregnancy.

D. **False.** These antibodies can cross the placenta and cause fetal thrombocytopenia. This needs to be considered when deciding on the most appropriate method of delivery.

44.

A. **False.** Diaphragmatic hernias occur in 1:2000 to 3000 births. Usually, the defect is on the left side. Stomach, colon and even spleen may enter the chest through the defect. The heart is pushed to the right, and the lungs may become hypoplastic.

B. **True.** Approximately 95 per cent of these fetuses are stillborn. Over 15 per cent of cases have associated abnormalities, and diaphragmatic hernia is associated with a number of syndromes, including Beckwith–Wiedeman syndrome, Pierre–Robin syndrome, Fryuse syndrome and chromosome defects such as trisomy 13, trisomy 18 and deletion of 9p syndrome.

45.

A. **False.**

B. **False.** Insulin requirements may increase slightly, but this is not an absolute contraindication.

C. **False.** The COCP reduces menstrual loss and risk of intraperitoneal haemorrhage at ovulation.

D. **False.** Low-dose pills are not associated with an increased risk of developing hypertension.

46.

A. **True.** Amiodarone is an anti-arrhythmic, which should be used only if there is no alternative. It may depress the fetal thyroid activity and cause neonatal goitre.

B. **True.** They adversely affect blood pressure and renal function in the fetus and the newborn. Skull defects and oligohydramnios are also possible.

C. **True.** Beta-blockers can also cause neonatal bradycardia and hypoglycaemia.

D. **True.** Methyldopa is widely used and thought to be safe. In high doses it may lead to ileus and it may give a false-positive result of the Coombs' test in the fetus.

47.

A.   **False.**   The incidence of breech presentation at term is said to be of the order of 3–4 per cent, and in those of birth weight less than 2.5 kg the incidence is 2.6–3.0 per cent. The incidence in the preterm pregnancy is high, and at 29–32 weeks' gestation is 25 per cent.

B.   **False.**   25 per cent.

C.   **False.**   Approximately 75 per cent of breeches convert spontaneously. The incidence of spontaneous version after 32 weeks may be as high as 57 per cent, and after 36 weeks' gestation may be as high as 25 per cent.

D.   **True.**   Spontaneous version is more likely in multiparous patients without a previous breech birth, and less likely in nulliparous women.

E.   **False.**   Cerebellar damage and ataxic cerebral palsy.

F.   **True.**   This is thought to contribute to the higher mortality and morbidity, even when delivered by the abdominal route.

48.

A.   **True.**

B.   **True.**   Preterm mortality rate is 25–30 per cent.

C.   **True.**   Unlike early onset where the majority of infections are vertically transmitted (birth canal).

D.   **True.**

E.   **True.**   Unlike early onset disease where the majority present with pneumonia as well as septicaemia.

F.   **True.**   As well as septic arthritis, osteomyelitis, empyema, endocarditis, cellulitis.

G.   **False.**   20 per cent.

H.   **True.**

49.

A.   **False.**   Steroids and aminophylline are the drugs of choice for a severe attack of asthma, and should not be withheld in pregnancy.

B.   **True.**   Pulmonary embolism can present with bronchospasm. Pulmonary embolism is more common in pregnant than in non-pregnant women.

C.   **False.**   The asthmatic mother has at least twice the chance of having a child who develops asthma.

D.   **False.**   Prostaglandin E_2 does have a vasoconstrictive effect on the bronchus, but in practice this is not usually a problem with careful induction.

Asthma with pregnancy

Incidence

About 1 per cent of all pregnancies are complicated by asthma, around 1 per cent of which will require admission to hospital. Of the patients with asthma who become pregnant, one-third will experience no change in their illness, just over half will worsen, and the remainder will improve. As far as the next pregnancy is concerned, two-thirds will experience a similar disease pattern.

Drugs used in pregnancy with asthma

The drugs used are essentially the same as those used in non-pregnant individuals:

- Bronchodilators, e.g. beta-agonists.
- Anti-inflammatory agents, e.g. steroids.
- Antibiotics, e.g. amoxicillin.

Although most medications have not been tested in pregnant populations, poorly controlled asthma has been associated with many complications, including low birth weight and complications of labour.

Features of pulmonary embolism

Clinical diagnosis of pulmonary embolism is often difficult. Post-mortem studies show it to be a very common condition (microemboli found in up to 60 per cent of all autopsies).

Symptoms include:

- Pleuritic pain.
- Cough with haemoptysis.
- Sudden-onset pallor and sweating.

Signs include:

- Dyspnoea, tachypnoea.
- Tachycardia.
- Prominent 'a' wave in the jugular venous pulse.
- Systolic and diastolic murmurs due to turbulent flow.
- Pleural rub.
- Pyrexia.

Investigations include:

- Chest X-ray (often normal).
- ECG – may show sinus tachycardia and, classically, S wave in lead I and Q wave and inverted T waves in lead III (S1, Q3, T3).
- Elevated serum D-dimer, although beware false positives.
- Pulmonary V/Q scan.
- Doppler ultrasound.

50.

A. **False.** Secondary PPH may occur at any time after the first 24 h following delivery until the 6 weeks of the puerperium are completed.

B. **True.** Most haemorrhages occur between 5 and 10 days after delivery. Secondary postpartum haemorrhage occurs following about 1 per cent of births.

C. **False.** PPH remains a significant cause of maternal mortality. In a recent Report on Confidential Enquiries into Maternal Deaths (*Why Mother's Die,* 2001), 11 of the 22 maternal deaths directly due to bleeding disorders presented with PPH.

D. **True.** According to recent meta-analyses, the need for blood transfusion is also reduced.

51.

A. **True.**

B. **True.**

C. **False.**

D. **False.**

52.

A. **True.** Duodenal atresia occurs in 1:7000 live births. The stomach and proximal duodenum distend to give the classic double-bubble appearance, which is associated with polyhydramnios. Jejunal atresia produces a triple-bubble appearance.

B. **True.** In 30 per cent of cases.

C. **False.** Oesophageal atresia occurs in 1:3000 live births. The double-bubble sign is present in one-third of the patients.

53.

A. **True.** Galactorrhoea is an associated finding in 30–80 per cent.

B. **True.** Thyrotrophin-releasing hormone is a stimulator of prolactin secretion.

C. **False.** Dopamine is an inhibitor of prolactin, therefore dopamine agonists (e.g. bromocriptine) reduce prolactin concentrations. The main control of prolactin secretion is inhibitory. Drugs that interfere with dopamine synthesis can increase prolactin levels.

D. **False.** Hyperprolactinaemia has no adverse effect in pregnancy. However, in patients with macroprolactinomas, bromocriptine should be used to normalize prolactin prior to pregnancy, but discontinued at the first sign of pregnancy.

E. **True.**

> ### Prolactin
>
> Prolactin is a monomeric polypeptide of 198 amino acids. Growth hormone and human placental lactogen are structurally similar to prolactin.
>
> At all times, the pattern of release is pulsatile – particularly during sleep. Prolactin secretion is regulated by a short negative feedback control system, hypothalamic prolactin inhibiting factor (PIF), which is probably dopamine.
>
> Increased secretion of prolactin is caused by stress, stimulation of nipple, exposure to oestrogens, thyrotrophin-releasing hormone (TRH), vasoactive intestinal peptide (VIP), epidermal growth factor and certain drugs, including dopamine antagonists (e.g. phenothiazines and metoclopramide).
>
> Bromocriptine, L-dopa and dopamine suppress prolactin secretion.

54.
A. **False.** It is 10–20 per cent over and above transmission occurring either *in utero* or at delivery.
B. **False.** Passively acquired maternal antibodies persist for up to 18 months, hampering serological diagnosis. An earlier diagnosis can be made by virus culture, polymerase chain reaction (PCR), the detection of p24 antigen, IgA or in-vitro antibody production tests, usually by 3 months of age.
C. **False.** One-quarter, often with *Pneumocystis carinii* pneumonia.
D. **True.** But it resolves with discontinuation of treatment.
E. **False.** Based on current knowledge, there is no justification for this policy.
F. **True.**

55.
A. **False.** Ectopic pregnancy is not a contraindication. Overall, the incidence of ectopic pregnancy is reduced by 50 per cent by IUCD.
B. **True.** The IUCD is not recommended for women who are at increased risk of bacterial endocarditis, or who have a history of endocarditis, rheumatic heart disease or the presence of prosthetic heart valves. Women with mixed mitral valve prolapse can use an IUCD, but antibiotic prophylaxis (amoxycillin 2 g) should be provided 1 h before insertion.
C. **True.** The IUCD is contraindicated in patients with a history of valvular heart disease.

56.
A. **False.** Usually first 24 h; mean age 20 h.
B. **True.**
C. **False.** Septicaemia or pneumonia, 30 per cent concomitant meningitis. Differentials: respiratory distress syndrome, transient tachypnoea of the newborn, congenital cardiac heart disease, hypoxic ischaemic encephalopathy.

57.
A. True.
B. True.
C. True.
D. True.

58.
A. **False.** They do cross the placenta, thus accounting for neonatal myasthenia gravis in 10–20 per cent of babies born to affected mothers.
B. **True.** Unfortunately, remission in the first 6 months of the postnatal period occurs in about 75 per cent of cases.

59.
A. **True.** Other side effects include diarrhoea, abdominal pain, dyspepsia, intermenstrual bleeding and menorrhagia.
B. **True.** Nausea, vomiting, diarrhoea, hyperthermia and flushing as with other prostaglandins.
C. **True.** Only with high doses and large volumes of electrolyte-free fluids.
D. **True.**
E. **True.** Nausea, vomiting, diarrhoea, hyperthermia and flushing as with other prostaglandins. Less commonly: hypertension, pulmonary oedema, chills, diaphoresis and dizziness.

60.
A. True.
B. True.
C. **True.** Alternatively, a rise in systolic pressure of >30 mmHg or a rise in diastolic pressure of >15 mmHg over the booking blood pressure.
D. **False.** 7–10 per cent.
E. True.

61.
A. **False.** The incidence of twins is 12:1000.
B. True.
C. True.
D. True.
E. **False.** The structural defects are usually confined to one twin, while the other is normal in 85–90 per cent of cases.
F. **False.** CVS is less appropriate as it is difficult to be sure that both placentas have been sampled, especially if they are lying close together.
G. **False.** The true figure is 50 per cent, despite the absence of obvious vaginal bleeding or miscarriage.
H. **True.** This is true, but it may reduce the rate of handicap.

> ### Multiple pregnancy
>
> Incidence:
>
> - World-wide incidence varies from 45:1000 in Nigeria to 4:1000 in Japan.
> - The incidence of monozygotic twinning is constant; the increased incidence is due to dizygous twins.
> - Perinatal mortality is four times that for singleton.
> - 40 per cent deliver before 37 weeks.
>
> The type of monozygotic twin pregnancy depends on the timing of separation of the embryo:
>
> - Up to 4 days: dichorionic, diamniotic (11 per cent).
> - 4–7 days: monochorionic diamniotic (22 per cent).
> - 7–14 days: monochorionic, monoamniotic (1 per cent).
> - More than 14 days: conjoined twins.
> - Dizygotic twins account for the other 66 per cent.

62.

A. **True.** Thromboembolism accounts for around 20 per cent of perioperative hysterectomy deaths (Department of Health, 1993). Patients undergoing gynaecological surgery should be assessed for clinical risk factors and overall risk of thromboembolism, and receive prophylaxis according to the degree of risk. This is highest for surgery associated with malignancy, less in abdominal hysterectomy, and lowest for vaginal hysterectomy. Patient risk factors include age over 40 years, obesity, previous DVT, blood group other than O, and the presence of congenital or acquired thrombophilias.

B. **True.** Although the use of low molecular-weight heparin is associated with a 5–15 per cent increase in the incidence of wound haematoma, there are no significant changes in postoperative haemoglobin levels or blood transfusion requirements.

C. **True.** It is estimated that the risk of postoperative thromboembolism is 0.96 per cent for low-dose pill users (<50 micrograms ethinyloestradiol) and 0.5 per cent for non-users. RCOG guidelines advise that the COCP need not be stopped routinely prior to procedure preformed, and that appropriate prophylaxis should be administered.

D. **False.** Recent studies do show an increased risk.

63.

A. **True.** The urinary bladder is composed of a syncytium of smooth muscle fibres known as the detrusor. The trigone is an easily distinguishable triangular area at the base of the bladder and is bounded by the ureteric orifices and the urethra. The normal bladder volume ranges from 450 to 600 mL.

B. **False.** The detrusor muscle is innervated by parasympathetic nerves S2–S4 and receives a rich efferents supply. Adrenergic receptors present in the lower urinary tract. Sympathetic outflow is from T10 to L2.

C. **True.** Anatomical factors in the maintenance of urinary continence include striated muscles of the pelvic floor, pubourethral ligaments, the external urethral sphincter and urethral smooth muscle, periurethral collagen and connective tissue and mucosal coaptation of the urothelium.

D. **False.** The normal maximum flow rate is 15 mL/s.

E. **False.** Stimulation of the parasympathetic nervous system and acetylcholine release is responsible.

Bladder filling:

- The normal bladder fills with only a small rise in intravesicular pressure: approximately 10 cm H_2O (above 15 cm H_2O is abnormal). This is the result of progressive relaxation of the detrusor smooth muscle, which occurs partly under the influence of the sympathetic nervous system.

- The sensation of bladder filling does not occur until a volume of 200 to 250 mL is reached, and the maximum capacity is 500–600 mL (when acute discomfort occurs). Voluntary voiding is controlled by the pontine micturition centre, which produces contraction of the detrusor muscle and simultaneous urethral relaxation; these continue until the contents of the bladder have been completely expelled, leaving a negligible residual volume.

64.

A. **True.**

B. **True.** Results from the MORE randomized trial. Cummings *et al.*, *JAMA* 1999; **281**: 2189–97.

C. **True.**

D. **False.**

E. **False.** May actually cause hot flushes.

The MORE Trial

A randomized trial in which 7705 women were assigned to receive raloxifene 60 mg/day, 120 mg/day, or placebo. The 4-year data showed that:

- Lumbar spine bone mineral density (BMD) was increased by 3.3 per cent from baseline and by 2.5 per cent compared to placebo for both 60 and 120 mg raloxifene (p <0.001).
- Femoral neck BMD was increased by 0.8 and 1.0 per cent from baseline and by 2.1 and 2.3 per cent compared to placebo for 60 and 120 mg raloxifene, respectively (p <0.001).
- Serum osteocalcin was decreased by 8.6, 26.2 and 31.1 per cent in the placebo, 60 and 120 mg raloxifene groups, respectively (p <0.001).
- The 4-year cumulative incidences of new vertebral fractures in the placebo, 60 and 120 mg raloxifene groups were 12.6, 8.0 and 7.2 per cent, respectively.
- The relative risks of new vertebral fractures were 0.64 (95% CI 0.53–0.76) for 60 mg and 0.57 (95% CI 0.48–0.69) for 120 mg raloxifene.

Raloxifene is licensed for prevention and treatment of postmenopausal osteoporosis. Unlike HRT, it does not reduce menopausal vasomotor symptoms. Raloxifene may reduce the incidence of oestrogen receptor-positive breast cancer, but its role in established breast cancer is not yet clear.

Side effects: venous thromboembolism, thrombophlebitis, hot flushes, leg cramps, peripheral oedema, influenza-like symptoms, rarely rashes and gastro-intestinal disturbances.

Dose: 60 mg once daily.

65.
A. **False.** Severe lupus nephropathy may worsen, but there is no reliable evidence to show that pregnancy in itself worsens SLE.
B. **True.** It is also associated with pregnancy loss and small-for-gestational-age fetuses.
C. **False.** Caesarean section is reserved for the usual obstetric indications.
D. **False.** Neonatal lupus erythematosus is characterized by congenital heart block, skin lesions, thrombocytopenia and haemolytic anaemia.
E. **True.** Many babies born with congenital heart block due to SLE are born to asymptomatic mothers.

66.
A. **True.** It allows ideal visualization of the tubal mucosa, but oil-based media obscures the detail of tubal anatomy.
B. **True.** Patients with a history of pelvic infection or demonstrating adnexal tenderness should receive an antibiotic course first.
C. **False.** It should be performed within 12 h of intercourse, and at mid cycle. The cervical mucus is assessed for quality, quantity and number of motile sperm.
D. **True.** Abundant clear, watery, relatively acellular cervical mucus should also be present.

67.
A. **True.** During the fifth menstrual week when it measures at least 10 mm.
B. **False.** First, a sac; then a yolk sac, followed by fetal pole and fetal heart.
C. **True.** Heart motion may be seen from 38 days.
D. **True.** From 6 to 9 weeks' gestation there is a rapid increase in the mean heart rate, from 125 to 175 bpm. Thereafter, the heart rate gradually decreases to around 160 bpm at 14 weeks.

Ultrasound features of pregnancy:

- thick endometrium   28 days;
- sac with double halo   32 days;
- yolk sac   36–40 days;
- fetal pole   38 days;
- fetal heart   40 days.

68.
A. **False.** Transient neonatal hypoglycaemia and body hair abnormalities (alopecia) have been reported with the use of diazoxide, as both an antihypertensive and a tocolytic agent.
B. **True.** Transient neonatal thrombocytopenia.
C. **True.** Subsequently, uteroplacental perfusion is decreased.
D. **False.**
E. **False.** Maternal use of frusemide seems to displace bilirubin from albumin, possibly causing neonatal hyperbilirubinaemia.

Causes of neonatal thrombocytopenia:

- Systemic maternal disease; idiopathic thrombocytopenia, systemic lupus erythematosus (SLE).
- Drugs; quinine or thiazides.
- Inherent platelet abnormality or defective platelet synthesis.
- Inherited metabolic disease; methylmalonic acidaemia.
- Marrow replacement; with leukaemia and neuroblastoma.

69.
A. **False.** Pneumonia occurs in approximately 10 per cent. Mechanical ventilation may be required, and mortality rates of up to 6 per cent have been reported.
B. **True.**
C. **False.** 2 per cent. The risk of spontaneous miscarriage after first-trimester varicella infection is not increased.

Congenital varicella syndrome

Symptoms:

• Skin scarring in a dermatomal distribution.

• Eye defects (microphthalmia, chorioretinitis, cataracts).

• Hypoplasia of the limbs.

• Neurological abnormalities (microcephaly, cortical atrophy, mental retardation, dysfunction of bowel and bladder sphincters).

70.

A. **False.** Polycystic ovaries remain active despite anovulation/oligoamenorrhoea, and substantial amounts of oestradiol continue to be produced. Risk no greater than for normal ovulatory women.

B. **True.** There is an increased risk of endometrial cancer into late adult life. Ovarian tissues remain active under influence of insulin beyond the menopause. Associated with nulliparity, diabetes mellitus and hypertension.

C. **False.** Late-onset adrenal enzyme deficiencies may be present in about 10 per cent of patients. 17-hydroxyprogesterone is a screening test, and adrenocorticotrophic hormone (ACTH) stimulation testing may be needed. Co-treatment with glucocorticoid is then used.

D. **True.** And lipid abnormalities.

E. **False.** The risk of non-insulin-dependent diabetes mellitus (NIDDM) is increased during pregnancy, treatment with sex steroids and late adult life.

71.

A. **True.**

B. **False.** The incidence of pain is less with interrupted sutures.

C. **False.** Polyglycolic acid sutures (e.g. Dexon, Vicryl) should be used in preference to glycerol-impregnated or other catgut or silk as they produce less short-term pain and require less use of analgesia.

Absorbable sutures

The use of absorbable synthetic material (Dexon and Vicryl) for the repair of perineal trauma is associated with less perineal pain, analgesic use, dehiscence and resuturing when compared with catgut suture material. The problem with Dexon and Vicryl is the length of time they take to be absorbed, as approximately 60 per cent remains for up to 21–28 days, and the material is not totally absorbed from the wound until 60–90 days. Vicryl Rapide, due to a sterilization process using gamma irradiation, maintains its tensile strength for just 10–14 days and it is therefore fully absorbed within 35–42 days. The use of a continuous subcuticular technique for perineal skin closure is associated with less short-term pain than techniques employing interrupted sutures.

72.
A. **False.** 30–35 per cent will die within 5 years of diagnosis.
B. **True.** Approximately 50 per cent of cases will be local recurrence, 30 per cent distant, and the remainder mixed.
C. **False.** Approximately one-third of cases occur within 1 year, but three-quarters occur within 3 years.
D. **True.** However, up to one-third of patients are often free of symptoms at the time the recurrence is detected.

73.
A. **True.** Obesity is associated with hyperinsulinaemia, and insulin suppresses the synthesis of sex hormone-binding globulin.
B. **True.** Hair cover is graded 0 to 4 on 11 defined body areas.
C. **True.** There are ethnic differences in the prevalence of, and attitudes to, hirsutism.
D. **False.** Up to 92 per cent of patients with idiopathic hirsutism have polycystic ovarian disease.

74.
A. **False.** It is about 10–25 per cent
B. **True.** Caffeine also may decrease fertility.
C. **False.** Severe endometriosis can structurally damage the anatomic relationship between tubes and ovaries, leading to decreased fertility.
D. **True.** Intermenstrual bleeding may be the only symptom of chlamydial cervicitis. Other causes of tubal disease are ruptured appendix, septic abortion, ectopic pregnancy, previous tubal surgery, intra-uterine contraceptive device and other sexually transmitted diseases.
E. **False.** The correct value is 30–40 per cent. Other factors include ovulatory dysfunction, pelvic disease and cervical factors, as well as unexplained problems.
F. **True.** Other factors associated with a poor pregnancy rate, even after tubal surgery, include severe pelvic adhesive disease, infertility after tuboplasty and endometriosis with tubal or ovarian involvement.

75.
A. **True.**
B. **True.** Due to polyhydramnios. Other risk factors are smoking, previous preterm labour, uterine abnormality, fetal demise, urinary tract infection, previous cervical surgery and chorioamionitis.
C. **True.** And 10 per cent of perinatal mortality.
D. **True.** The background rate is 7 per cent. In patients with previous preterm labour this rises to between 14 and 18 per cent.
E. **True.**
F. **True.** Such as placental abruption or acute polyhydramnios. Subclinical infection is thought to be an important aetiological factor in the remainder.
G. **False.** Phospholipase A_2 releases arachidonic acid from membrane-bound phosphatidylethanolamine and phosphatidylinositol, the first stage in prostaglandin E_2 (PGE_2) and prostaglandin F_2 (PGF_2) synthesis. Whilst unable to release phosphatidyglycerols (PGs) directly, as they lack cyclo-oxygenase and lipoxygenase, bacteria release phospholipase of higher specificity than endogenous phospholipase A_2 found in the membranes and deciduas.
H. **True.**

76.
A. **False.** Abortion, stillbirth and premature delivery are not increased. The disease for which the steroids are given is the main complication.
B. **False.** It is natural progesterone with no known adverse effects on the fetus.
C. **True.** Diethylstilbestrol (DES) in pregnancy has led to minor vaginal structural and epithelial abnormalities (adenosis), and also some cases of vaginal adenocarcinoma.
D. **True.** The 19 Nor-steroids (Norethisterone and Norgestrel) are derivatives of testosterone, and can cause masculinization of the female fetus.

Abnormalities in the offspring of pregnant women exposed to diethylstilbestrol (DES)

Female offspring: clear-cell adenocarcinoma of the vagina or cervix, vaginal adenosis, T-shaped uterus, uterine hypoplasia, paraovarian cyst or incompetent cervix. They are known as 'daughters of DES'. The National Maternity Hospital in Dublin runs a special DES clinic to review and colposcope these girls on a regular basis.

Male offspring: epididymal cyst, hypoplastic testes or cryptorchidism.

77.
A. **True.**
B. **False.** Autosomal recessive.
C. **False.** Autosomal dominant.
D. **True.**
E. **False.** Phenylketonuria is an autosomal recessive disorder, in which there is deficiency of the enzyme phenylalanine hydroxylase; this leads to low levels of tyrosine, and high (toxic) levels of phenylalanine.
F. **True.** It occurs in 1:10 000 live births. It is due to a 21-hydroxylase deficiency. It is associated with ambiguous genitalia in a female fetus or macrogenitosomia in a male fetus.
G. **True.** It is the commonest cause of mental retardation after Down's syndrome, and the commonest form of inherited mental handicap.
H. **True.** The incidence is 1:20 000 live births. The individual is tall, doliocephalic, and carries the risk of kyphoscoliosis, ectopia lentis, aortic regurgitation and dissecting aortic aneurysm.
I. **True.** It is caused by mutations in the dystrophin gene and affects 0.3:1000 males.
J. **True.** Von Willebrand's disease is due to deficiency of factor VIII carrier protein. It usually presents as a platelet disorder.
K. **False.** Thalassaemia is inherited in an autosomal recessive manner.

Inheritance of diseases

Autosomal dominant:

Adult polycystic kidney disease, familial hypercholesterolaemia, Huntington's disease, malignant hyperthermia, myotonic dystrophy, neurofibromatosis, tuberous sclerosis, von Hippel–Lindau disease.

Autosomal recessive:

Cystic fibrosis, thalassaemia, Tay–Sachs disease, sickle-cell disease, congenital adrenal hyperplasia, galactosaemia, mucopolysaccharidosis, phenylketonuria.

X-linked recessive:

Albinism, angiokeratoma, chronic granulomatous disease, ectodermal dysplasia, fragile X syndrome, haemophilia, ichthyosis, Lesch–Nyham syndrome, Menke's syndrome, muscular dystrophy (Duchenne's and Becker's), retinitis pigmentosa.

78.
A. **True.** This is thought to occur in 25 per cent of deliveries.
B. **True.** Haemorrhoids affect 18 per cent of women. They are more common in primiparous women and after assisted vaginal delivery.
C. **False.** In 26 of 27 cases in a recent report (*Why Mothers Die*), death occurred after delivery. Epidural analgesia in labour should not be relied upon by itself to control blood pressure. Ergometrine should not be used for the third stage in hypertensive women.

79.
A. **False.** Acyclovir may be expected to reduce the severity and duration of the illness, but there are theoretical concerns about teratogenesis when acyclovir is used in the first trimester.
B. **True.**
C. **False.** It should be administered intravenously. In certain circumstances it may be necessary to consider mechanical ventilation.

Acyclovir

Acyclovir is active against herpes viruses, but does not eradicate them. It is effective only if started at the onset of the episode. Uses of acyclovir include the systemic treatment of varicella-zoster (chickenpox-shingles) and the systemic and topical treatment of herpes simplex infections of the skin and mucous membranes (including initial and recurrent genital herpes). It can be life-saving in herpes simplex and varicella-zoster infections in the immunocompromised. Side effects include gastro-intestinal disturbance, headache, fatigue, rash, rarely hepatitis, jaundice, dyspnoea, angioedema, anaphylaxis, neurological reactions, acute renal failure and decreases in haematological indices.

On intravenous infusion, severe local inflammation, fever, and rarely agitation, tremors, psychosis and convulsions may occur.

80.

A. **False.** Neonatal hypothyroidism may occur if the mother is receiving antithyroid drugs (carbimazole or propylthiouracil) or carries antithyroid antibodies.

B. **True.** The hydantoin agents, phenytoin, ethotoin and mephenytoin, are well known for their association with a constellation of congenital anomalies known as the fetal hydantoin syndrome. Cardiac defects and diaphragmatic hernias have also been reported. Like phenobarbitone, there is an increased risk of neonatal haemorrhage; therefore vitamin K should be administered to the neonate at birth and the mother in late pregnancy.

C. **True.**

D. **False.** It is reported to be associated with an increased risk of neural tube defects, estimated to be in the range 1–2 per cent. In addition, there is an increased risk of microcephaly and cardiac abnormalities. Thus, it is advisable to give folic acid in the first trimester and preconceptionally (5 mg).

Features of the fetal hydantoin syndrome:

- Craniofacial abnormalities.
- Cleft lip/palate.
- Hypertelorism.
- Broad nasal bridge.
- Hypoplasia of distal phalanges and nails.
- Growth deficiency.
- Mental deficiency.

81.

A. **False.** The benefits of diagnosis far outweigh the risks.

B. **False.** Warfarin does not cross into the breast milk in significant quantities, because it is highly protein bound.

C. **False.** It can be given safely to breast-feeding mothers. However, this anticoagulant may result in adverse fetal effects such as intracerebral haemorrhage, microcephaly, cataracts, blindness and mental retardation when utilized during the second or third trimester of pregnancy.

D. **False.** Long-term use of heparin will lead to maternal osteoporosis.

E. **False.** Heparin does not cross the placenta and is not secreted into breast milk, as it is a mucopolysaccharide that is highly ionized at physiological pH.

F. **True.** Heparin may be reversed with protamine sulphate (1 mg/100 UI heparin), to a maximum of 50 mg.

Anticoagulant use during pregnancy and lactation

Heparin:

- During pregnancy: osteoporosis has been reported after prolonged use.
- During lactation: none reported.

Oral anticoagulants:

- During pregnancy: congenital malformations, fetal and neonatal haemorrhage.
- During lactation: risk of haemorrhage, increased by vitamin K deficiency; warfarin appears safe, but phenindione should be avoided.

82.

A. **False.** The risk is 1:4. The carrier rate in UK is 1:10 000.

B. **False.** Alpha-thalassaemia is often, but not always, due to a gene deletion defect, unlike beta-thalassaemia.

C. **False.** The haemoglobinopathies are inherited defects of haemoglobin resulting from impaired globin synthesis (thalassaemia syndromes) or structural abnormality of globin (haemoglobin variants).

D. **False.** The haemoglobin molecule consists of four globin chains (a, b, d, g), each of which is associated with a haem complex. There are three normal haemoglobins in man HbA, HbA2 and HbF – each of which contains two pairs of polypeptide globin chains. HbA (a2b2) should comprise over 95 per cent of the total circulating haemoglobin in the adult.

E. **False.** This is a variant of the beta globin chain.

F. **True.** Because renal complications result in a progressive inability to concentrate urine. This is due to sickling within the circulation of the renal medulla.

Haemoglobin in the fetus:

- Most haemoglobin in the fetus is HbF (alpha-2, gamma-2) and HbA2 (alpha-2, delta-2).

- HbF is resistant to denaturation by acid and alkali, and *in vivo* has a higher affinity for oxygen than adult haemoglobin.

- 90 per cent of fetal haemoglobin is HbF between 10 and 28 weeks of gestation. From 28–34 weeks a switch from (alpha-2, gamma-2) to (alpha-2, beta-2) begins.

- By term, the ratio of HbF to HbA is 80:20, and by 6 months only 1 per cent of haemoglobin is HbF (in a normal adult, <1 per cent of haemoglobin is HbF).

- Between 4–8 weeks the embryo manufactures some additional haemoglobins: Hb Gower 1, Gower 2 and Hb portland.

83.
A. **True.** Traditionally, hydrops has been considered under two headings – immune and non-immune. The evaluation and survival rates for the two differ markedly.
B. **True.** The incidence of new anti-D sensitization approximates 1:1000 births; the approximate incidence of old cases is 1.5:1000 births; the approximate incidence of sensitization from other antibodies is 3:1000.
C. **False.** The approximate incidence is 2–3 per cent of those women with either anti-D or other antibodies.
D. **False.** It has been estimated to be 9:1.
E. **False.** Without identifiable circulating antibodies to red blood cell (RBC) antigens.
F. **False.** Certain cardiovascular system abnormalities are amenable to therapy.
G. **False.** The reported mortality rates range between 50 and 90 per cent.

84.
A. **True.** This is due to hypoprothrombinaemia, because of malabsorption of vitamin K. The risk of obstetric haemorrhage is 10–20 per cent.
B. **False.**
C. **False.**
D. **False.** The correct figure is 40–60 per cent.
E. **True.**

Features of intrahepatic cholestasis:

- Pruritus is usually the initial symptom, and may be generalized. It frequently involves the palms and soles. This is followed by production of dark urine, but only a minority of patients develop jaundice.

- Insomnia and irritability are frequent complaints.

- There is no abdominal pain, anorexia, nausea or vomiting, and the liver is neither enlarged nor tender.

85.

A. **False.** Characteristics of malignant lumps include irregular borders and attachment to deep structures.

B. **False.** In general, lumps in women aged under 35 years are more likely to be benign. New lumps in women aged over 70 are more likely to be malignant.

C. **False.**

D. **True.**

E. **True.** Atypical hyperplasia displays the highest relative risk.

F. **True.** Bloody cyst aspirate should always be sent for cytological analysis.

86.

A. **True.**

B. **True.** As a consequence, raised serum urate levels are probably better regarded not as a diagnostic, predictive or specific indicator of pre-eclampsia, but as a sensitive indicator of impaired renal function and blood flow.

Blood pressure during normal pregnancy

Systolic blood pressure does not change in pregnancy; diastolic pressure is reduced in the first two trimesters and returns to the non-pregnant level at term.

87.

A. **True.** Other anticonvulsants cause competitive inhibition of prothrombin precursors. The affected factors are II, VII, IX and X.

B. **True.** Weakness and myotonia are exacerbated, especially in the third trimester.

C. **False.** On the contrary, the typical complication is polyhydramnios due to paralysis of fetal swallowing: this accounts for the increased risk of premature labour.

88.

A. **False.** Anaemia, cardiac failure and hypoproteinaemia occur in a large number of cases, with cardiac failure being the commonest cause.

B. **True.** Infective agents can cause severe fetal anaemia that may lead to hydrops. Human parvovirus B19, cytomeaglovirus (CMV) and toxoplasmosis have been implicated.

C. **True.** 15–30 per cent are idiopathic.

D. **True.** In 70–85 per cent of cases.

89.

A. **False.** The development of the breast bud is the first sign, and occurs at approximately 10–11 years of age.

B. **True.** The relevant time periods are 3 and 5 years.

C. **False.** Peak velocity is achieved before menarche, but growth continues for some years after menarche.

D. **False.** This syndrome exhibits precocious pubertal development.

Causes of precocious sexual development:

- Constitutional (the commonest), in which the signs of puberty usually appear in correct order.

- The premature release of gonadotrophins from the pituitary, which may be stimulated by the presence of some intracranial lesions, e.g. meningitis, encephalitis, cerebral tumours, third ventricle haematoma or McCune–Albright syndrome (cystic changes in the bones are combined with precocious puberty and café-au-lait spots on the child's skin).

90.

A. **False.** The correct description of the syndrome is haemolysis, elevated liver function tests and low platelets.

B. **False.** 4–12 per cent.

C. **False.**

Laboratory values used to diagnose the HELLP syndrome

Haemolysis:

- Abnormal peripheral smear; increased bilirubin; increased lactate dehydrogenase.

Elevated liver enzymes:

- Increased serum oxaloacetic transaminase (SGOT); increased serum glutamic pyruvic transaminase (SGPT); increased lactic dehydrogenase (LDH).

Low platelets:

- Platelet count $<100 \times 10^9$/L.

91.

A. **True.** Both conditions involve proteinuria, hypertension and multi-organ system dysfunction. Thus, pre-eclampsia and active nephritis present with similar clinical signs.

B. **True.** At least 50 per cent of patients with RA demonstrate improvement in their disease in at least 50 per cent of their pregnancies.

C. **False.** Conception is not affected, but about 15–25 per cent of pregnancies in women with RA end in miscarriage.

92.

A. **True.**

B. **True.**

C. **True.** Although rare, this is a significant hazard and patients should be asked if they have a latex sensitivity.

D. **True.** Transvaginal ultrasound is superior to digital examination of the internal os as the external os can sometimes be closed. A shortened cervix is also an important, albeit less significant risk factor.

93.
A. **False.** The cardiac lesions are congenital heart block and endocardial fibroelastosis.
B. **True.**
C. **True.** The haematological abnormalities include autoimmune haemolytic anaemia, leukopenia, thrombocytopenia and hepatosplenomegaly.
D. **False.**
E. **True.**

94.
A. **True.** Between 12 per cent and 15 per cent of clinically recognized pregnancies miscarry.
B. **True.** Accounting for about 50 000 admissions in the UK each year.
C. **True.**
D. **True.** The shape of the gestational sac and the presence of an intra-uterine haematoma have also been proposed as sonographic factors associated with early miscarriage.
E. **False.** It has been suggested that subchorionic haematomas in early pregnancy are associated with an increased risk of spontaneous miscarriage where the critical factor is the site of the haematoma, not the volume.

95.
A. **False.** While this is the drug of choice in eclampsia, it does not prevent all seizure activity.
B. **False.**
C. **False.**
D. **False.**
E. **True.**

Treatment of eclampsia

Eclampsia should be treated with intravenous magnesium sulphate, followed by a magnesium sulphate infusion to prevent further seizures.

Loading dose:

- 4 g (8 mL) $MgSO_4$ 50% diluted in 20 mL of 0.9% sodium chloride, given i.v. over 5–10 min.
- Repeat 2–4 g i.v. if seizures continue.

Maintenance dose:

1 g $MgSO_4$ per hour. Add 25 g (i.e. 50 mL of 50% $MgSO_4$) to 250 mL of 0.9% NaCl and infuse at a rate of 12 mL/h.

Therapeutic range: 2–4 mmol/L (4.0–8.0 mg/dL).

Dose alterations:

- Oliguria ($\leq$100 mL over 4 h) or urea >10 mmol/L: give 1 g/h maintenance dose and measure Mg levels more frequently.
- ALT >250 IU/L: measure Mg levels every 2–4 h.
- Mg level >4 mmol/L: decrease maintenance dose to 0.5 or 1 g/h, depending on level.
- Mg level <1.7 mmol/L: consider further 2-g i.v. bolus over 20 min. Increase maintenance dose to 2.5 g/h.
- Mg level 1.7–2.0 mmol/L: although this is strictly 'subtherapeutic', provided that the patient is stable and levels are not persistently <1.7 mmol/L, it is reasonable to continue with a 2 g/h maintenance dose.

Toxicity:

- Loss of patellar reflex, weakness.
- Nausea, feeling of warmth, flushing, weakness.
- Somnolence, double vision, slurred speech   Mg level 5 mmol/L.
- Muscle paralysis, respiratory arrest   Mg level 6.0–7.5 mmol/L.
- Cardiac arrest   Mg level >12 mmol/L.

96.
A. **True.** Supporting routine antenatal screening for HIV (with informed consent).
B. **False.** Oral treatment with metronidazole or clindamycin reduces the risk of preterm labour and premature rupture of membranes in the second trimester.

97.
A. **True.**
B. **True.**
C. **True.**

Screening group B *Streptococcus*

Approximately 1 in 3 of infants born to women with GBS will themselves be colonized, but only 0.3/1000 liveborn infants in the UK develop early-onset disease. Therefore, screening for GBS carriage is not justified. To prevent one case of early-onset neonatal disease, 3000 women would need to be screened, and up to 1000 treated.

98.
A. True.
B. True. The commonest cause is pregnancy, and this must always be considered in a woman of childbearing age.
C. True. As are many other drugs including antipsychotics and any drug stimulating prolactin secretion.

99.
A. False.
B. False.
C. False.
D. False.
E. False.

Double and ectopic ureters

Partial or complete duplication of the ureter results from early splitting of the ureteric bud. The kidneys do not completely separate as a result of the intermingling of the collecting tubules. An ectopic ureter is one that opens anywhere, but the trigone and ectopic ureters opening below the urethral sphincter mechanism usually become clinically and anatomically evident, producing continuous urinary incontinence.

100.
A. False. DNA virus.
B. True.
C. False. 48 h before the rash appears.
D. True. Although contact is common; 85 per cent of the adult population is seropositive for varicella-zoster IgG antibody.
E. True. Following the primary infection, the virus remains dormant but can be re-activated to cause a vesicular erythematous skin rash in a dermatomal distribution known as herpes zoster (HZ). There is a case report of congenital varicella syndrome in an immunocompromised woman with disseminated herpes zoster.
F. False. It appears to increase. Up to 50 per cent of fetuses are infected when maternal infection occurs 1–4 weeks before delivery, and one-third of these babies develop clinical varicella, despite high titres of passively acquired maternal antibody.
G. True. Babies with no clinical evidence of varicella infection at birth can develop HZ in infancy, consistent with primary infection.

DNA-containing viruses:

- Adenoviruses: respiratory tract infections, keratoconjunctivitis.
- Papovaviruses: Verrucae.
- Herpesviruses: herpes simplex, varicella-zoster, cytomegalovirus, infectious mononucleosis (Epstein–Barr virus), HHV-6.
- Poxviruses: smallpox, vaccinia, molluscum contagiosum.
- Hepadnaviruses: hepatitis B.

101.

A. **True.** The transformation zone may vary in location and may recede within the vagina after the menopause. In situations such as the latter, various instruments may be used to dilate the endocervical canal to allow inspection of the transformation zone.

B. **False.** The iodine stains the glycogen in mature cells. Thus, Schiller's positive area is one which does not stain with iodine.

C. **True.** Other features associated with malignancy include mosaic and punctate patterns and short pollarded vessels.

Transformation zone

The transformation zone (TZ) is a circumferential region of tissue between the vaginal (squamous) and endocervical (columnar) tissue. It is composed of columnar epithelium which has descended onto the ectocervix, although the border between the columnar and squamous epithelium is usually not finally defined until adult life.

102.

A. **True.** PAPS leads to both recurrent miscarriage and second-trimester loss.

B. **True.** 15 per cent of women with recurrent miscarriage have persistently positive tests for aPL. When these women are treated with low-dose aspirin (LDA; 75 mg/day), the live birth rate is increased to 40 per cent and further increased to 70 per cent when they are treated with LDA and heparin (preliminary results).

C. **True.** Prostacyclin formation is blocked, and thus there is relative excess of thromboxane, which causes vasoconstriction and thrombosis.

Antiphospholipid syndrome

This diagnosis requires confirmatory antibody testing in the presence of specified clinical criteria. The latter include: unexplained arterial or venous thrombosis, recurrent pregnancy loss (three or more consecutive first-trimester losses).

Autoimmune thrombocytopenia: the laboratory criteria are either lupus anticoagulant or moderate to high levels of IgG anticardiolipin antibodies.

103.

A. **True.** This should only be carried out with very careful monitoring. Daily injections and follicle stimulation monitored with ultrasound and serum oestradiol.

B. **True.** It is characterized by increased vascular permeability, which can lead to ascites, pleural effusion and, rarely, a pericardial effusion.

C. **False.** The syndrome is characterized by ovarian enlargement, ascites, hypercoagulation and haemoconcentration.

D. **True.** Haemoconcentration increases the risk of deep venous thrombosis.

Grades of ovarian hyperstimulation:

- Mild: abdominal bloating, mild pain, ovarian size usually <8 cm.
- Moderate: increased pain, nausea, diarrhoea, ovarian size usually 8–12 cm with ascites.
- Severe: clinical ascites, haemoconcentration (Hct >45%, white blood cells (WBC) >15 000/mL), oliguria, liver dysfunction, ovarian size usually <12 cm.
- Critical: tense ascites (Hct >55%, WBC >25 000/mL), renal failure, thromboembolic phenomena.

104.

A. **True.** And a 2-h glucose ≥8 and ≤11 mmol/L.

B. **False.** The figure is 10 per cent.

C. **True.** This was the number found after 24 years of follow-up.

D. **True.** As long as IGT does not develop into diabetes mellitus, the fetus is probably not at an increased risk of intra-uterine death.

E. **True.** With measurement of the blood glucose concentration 1 h later.

Indications for glucose tolerance test:

- History of diabetes in a first-degree relative.
- Glycosuria on two or more occasions (second specimen after fasting).
- Maternal weight >90 kg.
- Previous baby weighing >4.5 kg.
- Previous unexplained intra-uterine death or nearly neonatal death.

105.

A. **True.** The vas deferens may be absent.

B. **True.** Could be due to drugs, alcohol or varicocele.

106.

A. **False.** The following conditions are aggravated: scleroderma, portal hypertension and neurofibromatosis, but not sarcoidosis.
B. **True.**
C. **True.**
D. **True.**
E. **False.** Most patients with Hodgkin's disease in pregnancy are asymptomatic and healthy.

Sarcoidosis

Sarcoidosis is a multisystem granulomatous disorder which usually affects young adults. The prevalence in the UK population (male and female) is approximately 19 in 100 000, with a female preponderance. It presents most commonly with respiratory symptoms or chest X-ray abnormalities (30 per cent), e.g. bilateral hilar lymphadenopathy.

107.

A. **False.**
B. **True.** A meta-analysis of histopathological findings of the endometrium in women with premenstrual bleeding showed a normal endometrium in 57 per cent of cases.
C. **True.** 13.1 per cent.
D. **True.**
E. **False.** Less than 10 per cent.

108.

A. **False.** 10 cm (4 inches) of cream is required. The diaphragm should be inserted no longer than 6 h before sexual intercourse. About a teaspoonful of spermicide cream or jelly should be placed in the dome prior to insertion. Some of the spermicide should be spread around the rim. The diaphragm should be left in place for approximately 6 h (but no more than 24 h) after coitus.
B. **False.** The diaphragm by itself has little contraceptive effect, and its function is to maintain a high concentration of spermicide at the cervical entrance. Additional spermicide should be placed in the vagina before each additional episode of sexual intercourse while the diaphragm is in place.
C. **True.** It protects against ascending infection, and possibly also to some extent against intra-epithelial neoplasia.
D. **False.** The diaphragm is available in sizes from 50 to 105 mm diameter, in increments of 2.5–5 mm.

109.

A. **True.** Albumin 10 mg and b_2 microglobulin 1–2 mg.
B. **True.**
C. **False.** False-positive in the presence of alkaline urine, contamination with ammonia compounds, chlorhexidine or vaginal discharge, or in the presence of infection.
D. **True.**
E. **True.**

110.

A. **True.** This is a well-recognized risk factor.

B. **False.** Oligohydramnios is a recognized complication.

C. **True.** The exception to this is when the antihypertensives are associated with congenital anomalies. Angiotensin-converting enzyme (ACE) inhibitors are contraindicated in pregnancy.

D. **True.** Other complications include abruption and stillbirth.

ACE inhibitors

Angiotensin-converting enzyme (ACE) inhibitors block the conversion of angiotensin I to angiotensin II. They should be avoided throughout pregnancy. They may cause fetal abnormality such as skull defects. Later on, they may cause oligohydramnios and can affect renal function and blood pressure control in both the fetus and neonate.

111.

A. **True.** A clearer relationship between age and fecundity exists in men than in women.

B. **True.**

C. **True.** It affects 10–15 per cent of couples of reproductive age (i.e. aged 15–44 years).

D. **True.** Normal volume is >2 mL and pH of 7.2–7.8.

E. **True.** Normal morphology should be present in more than 50 per cent of cases.

Semen analysis

Normal values of semen analysis (according to WHO):

- Volume: ≥ 2.0 mL.
- Sperm concentration: $\geq 20 \times 10^6$/mL.
- Motility: ≥ 50 per cent with forward progression, or ≥ 25 per cent with rapid progression within 60 min of ejaculation.
- Morphology: ≥ 30 per cent normal forms.
- White blood cells: $< 1 \times 10^6$/mL.
- Immunobead test: <20 per cent spermatozoa with adherent particles.
- SpermMar test: <10 per cent spermatozoa with adherent particles.

112.

A. **True.** Pregnancy and lactation cause stress to maternal calcium homeostasis.

B. **False.** Total maternal calcium and phosphate concentrations decrease in pregnancy, but maternal ionized calcium remains unchanged.

C. **True.** The gradient is thought to be controlled by parathyroid hormone-related peptide, which probably originates in the fetal parathyroid glands and is stored in the placenta.

113.
A. **True.**
B. **True.**
C. **True.**
D. **True.**
E. **False.** Subepithelial lymphocyte infiltration.

Dystrophy

Dystrophy means a disorder of structure or function due to altered nutrition (atrophy, hypertrophy or hyperplasia).

Lichen sclerosis is one of the vulval dystrophies which include hyperplastic dystrophy and mixed atrophy which includes areas both thick and thin in their appearance.

Histologically, lichen sclerosus shows not only a thin and inactive epithelium, but also hyperkeratosis, loss of elastic tissue, hyalinization of collagen layer and subepithelial infiltration with leukocytes. Extravasated blood cells are commonly seen.

114.
A. **True.** Of those that are malignant, most occur in women aged over 45 years.
B. **False.** Typically, polycystic ovaries are enlarged with thickened, white, sclerotic capsules and subcapsular follicular cysts of varying size. However, they may occasionally be normal in size.
C. **True.** Other conditions in which it is elevated include ovarian malignancy, menstruation and pelvic infection.
D. **True.** Torsion is twice as common on the right side.
E. **False.** Most cases occur in the reproductive years.

115.
A. **True.** The arrest occurs in the diplotene phase. Growth occurs independently of gonadotrophin stimulation.
B. **True.** This happens as the first meiotic division is completed.
C. **False.** Ovulation occurs 34–36 h after the start of the LH surge, and 10–12 h after the peak.
D. **False.** Prostaglandin levels are maximal just before menstruation. They may be important in initiating menstrual flow.

116.
A. **False.** Postnatal perineal pain occurs in 42 per cent of women after delivery. It persists beyond the first 2 months in 8–10 per cent after spontaneous vaginal delivery.
B. **True.** 8–10 per cent of patients will experience this.
C. **False.** Neither ultrasound nor megapulse have any clinical effect on perineal pain or bruising.

Perineal pain

In the UK, approximately 23–42 per cent of women will continue to have pain and discomfort for 10–12 days postpartum, and 8–10 per cent of women will continue to have long-term pain (for 3–18 months following delivery). In addition, 23 per cent of women will experience superficial dyspareunia at 3 months, 3–10 per cent will report faecal incontinence, and up to 19 per cent will have urinary incontinence.

117.
A. **True.**
B. **False.** The reverse is **True.**
C. **False.** The reverse is **True.**
D. **True.** Breast-feeding may have a more pronounced negative effect on bone density than pregnancy itself.

Pregnancy and bone density:

- Pregnancy causes bone demineralization in women with a previously normal skeleton.

- The trabecular (spine-like) bone is more affected by pregnancy and by heparin than cortical bone (hip-like).

- A small number of pregnant women will have osteoporotic consequences; pregnancy is a stress that unmasks a defective maternal skeleton. There is a net negative effect on bone mineral density with breastfeeding, despite calcium supplementation.

118.
A. **False.** In low-risk labours, intermittent auscultation is thought to be sufficient and more acceptable to the mother.
B. **False.** By nature, there is trauma to the fetal scalp and thus any history or suspicion of coagulation disturbance should be taken into account before such a device is used.

119.
A. **False.** The finding of high mid-pregnancy levels of MSAFP in the absence of fetal structural abnormality indicates an increased risk of intra-uterine growth restriction and death, oliohydramnios, placental abruption and preterm delivery.
B. **True.** High levels of MSAFP can perhaps be seen as an early manifestation of the sick placenta syndrome, which leads to diminished adhesiveness later.
C. **False.** High mid-pregnancy levels of MSAFP indicate an increased risk of later complications, which include intra-uterine growth restriction, preterm labour, and in at least one study, placental abruption.

120.
A. **False.** The opposite is true – these cells signify an adequate sample.
B. **False.** The correct solution is 95 per cent ethyl alcohol. Immersion in this solution should occur immediately after the smear is taken.
C. **False.** The cellular changes inherent to both overlap. Studies show similar rates of disease progression.

121.
A. **True.** The most effective regimen is a combination of EE with CPA. CPA is also a strong progestogen.
B. **False.** 35 micrograms EE and 2 mg CPA.
C. **True.**
D. **False.** This regimen gives effective contraception, essential when prescribing anti-androgens, and regularizes the menstrual cycle.
E. **True.** Treatment should be continued for at least 6 months, with a maximal effect around 18 months. Thereafter, the dosage can be weaned down or changed to the combined oral contraceptive pill (choosing a non-androgenic progestogen).

122.
A. **True.** The terms are synonymous.
B. **True.** Chronic stimulation of the ovary by elevated LH results in this appearance.
C. **False.** The mode of inheritance in relevant cases is X-linked dominant.
D. **False.** Analysis of families shows preferential transmission through the maternal line in keeping with intra-uterine modulation of a genetic susceptibility. Of note, this is identical to the mode of inheritance postulated for non-insulin-dependent diabetes mellitus.
E. **False.** The LH:FSH ratio is increased, i.e. the normal value is 1.5:1 and in PCOS it is 3:1.
F. **True.** Evidence of dysfunction within both the pituitary and the ovary gave rise to the hypothesis of a self-perpetuating vicious cycle. Hypersecretion of LH relative to FSH induces hyperactivity of ovarian stromal tissues, atresia of antral follicles and disordered ovarian steroidogenesis, and the resulting acyclical production of oestrogenic steroids in turn accentuates the hypersecretion of LH by the anterior pituitary.
G. **False.** PCOD is characterized by elevated serum concentrations of pituitary-derived LH and ovarian-derived hyperandrogenaemia.
H. **False.** LH is secreted by the anterior pituitary.
I. **False.** It is the same as non-insulin-dependent diabetes mellitus.
J. **True.**

123.
A. **False.** The true definition involves the said increase for at least 15 s.
B. **True.** Late decelerations are attributed to decreased uterine blood flow. Low oxygen tension is detected by chemoreceptors, causing parasympathetic stimulation and increased vagal activity, leading to a decrease in fetal heart rate.
C. **True.** Examples include entanglement of the umbilical cord around the fetal body, a true knot in the cord and cord prolapse. Thus, management is directed at relieving cord compression, e.g. change of maternal posture, facial oxygen and vaginal examination to rule out cord prolapse.

124.
A. **True.** Contrary to previous thinking, the haemoglobin levels for both twins are often not discordant.
B. **False.** In a twin pregnancy with one fetal loss in the third trimester, commonly labour is precipitated and 90 per cent of cases will deliver within 3 weeks.
C. **False.** This is true for the donor twin.
D. **False.** This is true if the second twin is the smaller.

Twin-to-twin transfusion syndrome (TTTS):

- Complicates up to 35 per cent of monochorionic multiple pregnancies.
- Accounts for 15 per cent of perinatal mortality in twins.
- The recipient develops polyhydramnios with raised amniotic pressure.
- The donor develop oligohydramnios, oliguria and growth restriction.
- Haemoglobin levels are often not discordant.
- The diagnosis is based on amniotic fluid and growth discordance.

Twin reversed arterial perfusion (TRAP) sequence: the donor twin is normal but it feeds a parasitic acardiac, acephalic second twin. It is possible that vanishing twin, TRAP sequence and TTTS all have similar aetiology, but occur at different gestational age.

125.
A. **True.** The incidence is 3 per cent: 1 per cent from placenta praevia, 1 per cent from abruptio placenta, and 1 per cent from other causes.
B. **False.** Vaginal examination, by speculum or digit, must be avoided until placenta praevia has been excluded.
C. **False.** 10 per cent of patients.

126.
A. **False.** The respiratory rate increases and dyspnoea, even on mild exertion, is a normal feature in late pregnancy.
B. **False.** The diuresis, which commences after delivery, and the consequent reduction in plasma volume, contributes to the initial fall in cardiac output.
C. **True.** Heart murmurs are frequently detected during pregnancy as a result of haemodynamic changes, such as a 50 per cent increase in blood volume. A third heart sound may also be heard.
D. **False.** Plasma volume begins to expand within a few weeks after conception. By 15 weeks there is an increase of about 50 per cent. It reaches a plateau between the 28th and 35th weeks of gestation.

Physiology of pregnancy

Respiratory function changes during pregnancy:

- Ventilation rate and tidal volume: increased.
- Respiratory rate and vital capacity: unchanged.
- Expiratory reserve and residual volume: decreased.

Normal auscultatory findings in pregnancy:

- Prominent S1.
- Split S1 (due to early mitral valve closure).
- Wider split S1 (common).
- S4 (rare).
- Systolic murmur (90%).

127.
A. **False.** Not Northern Ireland. Abortion remains a very grey area in Northern Ireland. The last act relating to abortion was the 1861 Offences against the Person Act amended by the 1945 Criminal Justice Act.
B. **True.**
C. **True.**
D. **False.** Two independent doctors who should not work together.

Certificate A: 'The Blue Form'

The certificate must be completed before an abortion is performed under Section1(1) of the Abortion Act 1967.

The five grounds for abortion listed on the form are:

1. The continuance of the pregnancy would involve risk to the life of the pregnant woman greater than if the pregnancy were terminated.
2. The termination is necessary to prevent grave permanent injury to the physical or mental health of the pregnant woman.
3. The pregnancy has NOT exceeded its 24th week, and that continuance of the pregnancy would involve risk, greater than if the pregnancy were terminated, of injury to the physical or mental health of the pregnant woman.
4. The pregnancy has NOT exceeded its 24th week, and that the continuance of the pregnancy would involve risk, greater than if the pregnancy were terminated, of injury to the physical or mental health of any existing child(ren) of the family of the pregnant woman.
5. There is a substantial risk that if the child were born it would suffer from such physical or mental abnormalities as to be seriously handicapped.

128.
A. **False.** Any type of sperm (sperm head, immotile sperm, defective sperm) can be injected. Sperm capacitation and acrosome reaction are unnecessary for successful fertilization.
B. **True.** Sperm can be aspirated from the vas deferens, epididymis or testis and used to fertilize an egg, using a micropipette.

129.
A. **True.**
B. **True.**
C. **False.**
D. **False.** Ovarian metastases occur in approximately 7 per cent of cases.
E. **False.**

130.
A. **False.** Placental abruption is the premature separation of a normally sited placenta. The incidence varies from 0.49 to 1.8 per cent.
B. **True.** In the remainder, haemorrhage is described as concealed.
C. **False.** Bleeding is characteristically dark and non-clotting.
D. **True.**
E. **False.** It commonly comes from maternal blood, but not always and not entirely in all cases.
F. **True.** With a history of one pregnancy complicated by placental abruption, the recurrence rate is estimated to be 5–16 per cent. Two consecutive abruptions increase the rate to 25 per cent.

131.
A. **False.** Barrier contraception is advised.
B. **False.** No direct relationship has been established between tamoxifen and spontaneous abortion, birth defects and fetal deaths, although these have all been reported.
C. **True.**
D. **True.** So it can stimulate the endometrium and cause endometrial tumours.
E. **False.** Although less than 10 per cent of receptor-negative tumours will respond.

132.
A. **True.**
B. **False.** About 18 per cent in women and 6 per cent in men.
C. **False.** The bone mineral density (BMD) is normal if it is within 1 standard deviation (SD) of a young normal adult (T-score above –1). Low bone mass or osteopenia: if BMD is between 1 and 2.5 SD below a young normal adult (T-score between –1 and –2.5). Osteoporosis: if BMD is 2.5 SD or more below a young normal adult (T-score at or below –2.5).

133.

A. **False.** The causes of placenta praevia are frequently unclear. The condition is more commonly encountered in older multiparous women, those with multiple pregnancies, and those who have previously been delivered by Caesarean section.

B. **False.** The incidence of placenta praevia is 1 in 100 pregnancies.

C. **True.** There have been several suggestions that fetal growth restriction is more commonly encountered in association with placenta praevia. The explanation is poor placenta function in the inhospitable lower segment.

D. **True.** The explanation being poor placenta function in the inhospitable lower segment.

E. **False.** The exact aetiology of placenta praevia is unknown, but various risk factors have been identified. These include age, parity and previous Caesarean section. A single Caesarean section scar increases the risk by 0.65 per cent, three scars by 2.2 per cent, and 4+ scars by 10 per cent.

F. **False.**

G. **False.** The maternal mortality in the developed world is 0.03 per cent.

H. **True.** Vaginal ultrasound is the best method of diagnosis and has been shown to be safer and more sensitive than abdominal ultrasound.

134.

A. **False.** The correct figure is between 4 and 26 per cent.

B. **True.** As many as 13 per cent of women develop a degree of faecal incontinence after their first vaginal delivery. Forceps delivery is associated with a significantly increased risk (up to eight-fold) of mechanical anal sphincter injury and altered faecal continence. Childbirth-related faecal incontinence is not rare, may become symptomatic immediately after delivery, and is frequently under-reported.

C. **False.** These deliveries are contraindicated in the presence of an incompletely dilated cervix, even though some have advocated the use of the vacuum extractor at 9–10 cm cervical dilatation. The operator should be experienced in its use and be willing to abandon the technique if progressive descent does not occur.

135.

A. **False.** Rheumatic fever is the most common aetiological agent in pregnant women with heart disease world-wide. The incidence of rheumatic heart disease has fallen in most countries because of antibiotics used to treat streptococcal infection.

B. **False.** Increased due to improvement in the management of children with these anomalies.

C. **False.** The number of maternal deaths in the UK associated with cardiac disease declined steadily until 20 years ago, but since then has remained static at approximately 0.2 per cent.

D. **True.** Especially tight mitral stenosis or an arteriovenous shunt, as it may precipitate pulmonary oedema.

E. **False.** Oral contraception or condoms are preferable. A coil may cause bacterial endocarditis, and antibiotic prophylaxis is required during insertion.

F. **False.** Beta-blocking drugs may cause fetal bradycardia, neonatal hypoglycaemia and, possibly, intra-uterine growth restriction. Their use is reserved to control angina or arrhythmia.

G. **False.** In Eisenmenger's complex an interventricular septal defect is associated with pulmonary hypertension, right ventricular hypertrophy and ultimately a right-to-left shunt. In addition, there is dextrorotation of the aorta overlying the septal defect and, when the tetralogy of Fallot is present, pulmonary artery stenosis.

Cardiac disease in pregnancy

The incidence of significant cardiac disease in pregnancy is <2 per cent (10–15 per cent if the mitral valve is included). Maternal mortality occurs in <1 per cent (up to 50 per cent with primary pulmonary hypertension and Eisenmenger's syndrome). The risk of fetal development of congenital heart disease is 10–24 per cent if maternal or parental congenital heart disease is present (more with maternal).

Heart disease still has potential for danger in pregnancy, although the patterns of such disease have changed. The most common problems involved in maternal death in modern times are cardiomyopathy (including puerperal type), dissecting thoracic aortic aneurysm and myocardial infarction. Pulmonary vascular disease carries a particularly high risk of death in pregnancy, e.g. 30–50 per cent in pulmonary hypertension. (*Why Mothers Die*)

Beta-blocking drugs:

Action is by competitive inhibition of catecholamines at beta-1 and beta-2 adrenoreceptors. The lipid-soluble drugs within this group (including propranolol and metoprolol) have a shorter half-life than atenolol. As concerns exist regarding fetal growth retardation and neonatal effects, it is suggested that the use of beta-blockers is reserved for women where methyldopa has not provided satisfactory control. (*Dewhurst's Textbook of Obstetrics and Gynaecology for Postgraduates,* 6th edn)

136.

A. **False.** Only 30 per cent of exomphalos are associated with chromosomal abnormalities, especially trisomy 18 (Edward's syndrome).

B. **False.** *Exomphalos* is an anterior abdominal wall defect as a result of failure of the gut to return to the abdominal cavity at 8 weeks' gestation. The hernia sac is covered by peritoneum and may contain both liver and intestine. In *gastroschisis* the abdominal wall defect is usually to the right and below the insertion of the umbilical cord. Small bowel (without peritoneal covering) protrudes and floats free in the peritoneal fluid.

C. **False.** The association is very small between gastroschisis and chromosomal abnormalities and is probably <1per cent. Gut atresia or stenosis may occur in 7–30 per cent. Cardiac lesions have been reported in 0–8 per cent of fetuses, but they tend to be minor and not demonstrated by ultrasound.

D. **False.** Ectopia vesica and ectopia cardia are associated with exomphalos: thus, it is vital to visualize the fetal bladder.

137.

A. **True.** This triad occurs in the third trimester. Blood pressure is considered increased if the systolic reading is >140 mmHg or the diastolic reading is >90 mmHg. Pregnancy-induced hypertension may be defined as a rise in systolic pressure >30 mmHg or diastolic pressure >15 mmHg over the patient's baseline blood pressure. Proteinuria is defined as >500 mg/24 h.

B. **False.**

C. **False.** Hypertensive disease in pregnancy occurs in 6–8 per cent of all live births. Nulliparity, extremes of reproductive age (<15 and >35 years of age), black race, history of pre-eclampsia in a first-degree female relative, diabetes, chronic hypertension, multiple gestations, and hydrops (isoimmunized or non-immune) are all recognized as risk factors.

D. **False.** The definition of severe pre-eclampsia is systolic blood pressure >160 mmHg and/or diastolic blood pressure >110 mmHg on two occasions at least 6 h apart, proteinuria (>5 g/24 h), oliguria (<500 mL/24 h), cerebral or visual symptoms, epigastric pain, pulmonary oedema, low platelets, increased liver function tests, or intra-uterine growth restriction.

E. **True.** We know that hypertension, proteinuria, and oedema are merely the signs and symptoms required for diagnosis of a systemic illness characterized by vasoconstriction and hypovolaemia. Organs, including the fetoplacental unit, show evidence of poor perfusion.

F. **False.** Some studies claim that smoking can be considered as a protective factor against pre-eclampsia.

> **Pre-eclampsia risk factors include:**
> - Nulliparity.
> - Maternal age less than 15 or more than 35 years.
> - Black race.
> - History of pre-eclampsia in a first-degree relative.
> - Chronic hypertension.
> - Chronic renal disease.
> - Diabetes mellitus.
> - Multiple gestation.
> - Hydrops.

138.
A. **False.** The normal hormonal changes probably account for the majority of cases.
B. **False.** Steroids have been shown to be of use in severe cases.
C. **True.** Due to hypocalcaemia.
D. **True.** And other cerebellar signs such as nystagmus due to Wernicke's encephalopathy from vitamin B6 deficiency.

139.
A. **False.**
B. **False.** A meta-analysis of trials of prophylactic antibiotics at the time of Caesarean section has shown that they are both effective and cost-effective. The risk of serious wound infection is decreased significantly.
C. **True.** Furthermore, all types of injury to the head and face of the baby (apart from cephalhaematoma) are more common after forceps delivery.
D. **False.** The use of ventouse compared with forceps is associated with a higher incidence of cephalhaematoma.
E. **False.** No significant differences have been shown between the two methods for low Apgar scores, or in the long-term follow-up of mothers and children.

140.
A. **True.** Although it can occur in all age groups.
B. **False.** Classically the vulva is white and shrunken.
C. **True.** Burying the clitoris and shrinking of the introitus.
D. **True.**
E. **False.** It may affect skin anywhere on the body. However, the commonest sites are the vulva, perineum, neck, shoulders and forearms.
F. **False.** 20 per cent of lesions occur in skin such as the thighs, buttocks, trunk or shoulders.
G. **False.** The risk is estimated to lie between 0 and 10 per cent with an average rate of 3 per cent.

Non-neoplastic epithelial disorders of skin and mucosa:

- Lichen sclerosus.
- Squamous cell hyperplasia (not otherwise specified).
- Other dermatoses including lichen simplex chronicus, lichen planus, psoriasis, dermatitis and eczema.

141.

A. **True.** Nulliparity is found in 41.8 per cent of cases of postmenopausal bleeding and endometrial carcinoma.

B. **False.** Early menarche (less than 10 years) carries a probability of 80 per cent. A meta-analysis found that a late menopause (more than 55 years), in association with postmenopausal bleeding carries a probability of having endometrial carcinoma of 45.5 per cent.

C. **False.** The incidence is decreased in COCP users.

D. **True.** Hypertension in association with postmenopausal bleeding carries a probability of having endometrial cancer of 30.7 per cent.

E. **False.**

142.

A. **False.** It is now more common to find the infective agent to be a coliform, such as *Escherichia coli* or another Gram-negative organism such as *Bacteroides fragilis*. The most virulent organism, which may cause postpartum pelvic infection, is a beta-haemolytic *Streptococcus*.

B. **True.**

C. **True.** In a recent government report there was a marked increase in deaths associated with genital tract sepsis. The majority of deaths occurring in this area were after Caesarean section.

143.

A. **True.** IUCDs are more likely to lead to sterility in nulliparous patients. However, it is worth remembering that infections that occur 3–4 months after insertion are due to acquired sexually transmitted diseases, and not the direct result of the IUCD. Pelvic inflammatory disease (PID) is extremely rare beyond the first 20 days after insertion.

B. **False.** The perforation rate varies between 0.6 and 1.3 per 1000 insertions (WHO 1997).

> ## Side effects of IUCD:
> - Perforation of the uterus or cervix, displacement or expulsion of the device, exacerbation of pelvic infection, heavy menses, dysmenorrhoea, allergy.
> - On insertion: pain (alleviated by non-steroidal anti-inflammatory drugs (NSAIDs) such as ibuprofen 30 min before insertion) and bleeding, occasionally, epileptic seizure, vasovagal attack.

144.
A. True. 13/1000.
B. True.
C. True.
D. True.
E. True.

145.
A. True.
B. False. IBS is a functional disorder of the bowel.
C. True. It is a very common condition and affects one-fifth of the general population.
D. True. However, no physical abnormality can be found at sigmoidoscopy, colonoscopy, ultrasound or barium enema.
E. True. Many drugs have been used, including antispasmodics and bulking agents. Most benefit is obtained from patient education, dietary advice and psychotherapy.
F. False. Symptoms suggestive of IBS include relief of pain with defaecation, episodes of pain more than once monthly, diarrhoea/constipation or the alternation of these, abdominal distension associated with acute exacerbation.

146.
A. False. This problem occurs in 8–9 per cent of vaginal breech deliveries. It happens because the abdomen and thorax deliver through an incompletely dilated cervix and are followed by the unmoulded head.
B. False. The main causes of increased perinatal mortality in breech presentations are hypoxia, congenital anomalies, prematurity and birth injury.
C. True. This occurs in 3–5 per cent of vaginal breech deliveries. The fetus is termed 'star-gazing'.
D. False. If the membranes are left intact for as long as possible, it is thought to prevent cord prolapse and to encourage cervical dilatation.
E. False. Vaginal delivery is advantageous to the fetus in several respects; among these are fewer respiratory problems and fewer complications due to iatrogenic prematurity.

147.

A. **False.** Turner's syndrome (XO) occurs in 1:3000 live births. The incidence is increased with increasing paternal age and decreased with increasing maternal age.

B. **True.** Early spontaneous loss of the fetus occurs in 95 per cent of cases.

C. **True.** Severely affected fetuses who survive to the second trimester can be detected by ultrasound and may show cystic hygroma, chylothorax ascites and hydrops.

D. **False.** Overall, 60 per cent of Turner's syndrome is due to pure XO, more are mosaics (usually XO/XX), and the rest are due to deletions, rings or isochromosomes of Xq or Xp.

E. **True.** In liveborn infants chromosomal abnormalities occur at about 6:1000. The incidence of autosomal and sex chromosome abnormalities is about the same.

F. **True.** The phenotype and fertility of XXX syndrome are normal and the abnormality frequently goes unnoticed, but there is an increased risk of sex chromosome abnormalities (4 per cent) and premature menopause of their offspring.

G. **False.** XXY (Klinefelter's syndrome) occurs in 1:700–1000 live births, and the rate increases with increasing maternal age.

H. **True.** The risk of breast cancer is also increased. Intelligence is generally in the normal range, but there are behavioural and educational problems.

I. **False.** Hypogonadism is the primary feature and azoospermia is the rule.

J. **False.** XXXX is an Australian beer. Nothing to do with sex chromosomal abnormalities. The real exam throws in a few googlies too: not usually as obvious as this one!

Turner's syndrome

Most XO conceptuses are early lethals. At birth, the incidence is 1 in 5000. This does not include the XO/XX mosaics or individuals with partial deletion of one X.

Typical features include small stature and tendency to obesity, ovarian dysgenesis, transient congenital lymphoedema, broad chest with wide-spaced nipples, abnormal auricles, narrow maxilla, small mandible, low posterior hairline and webbed neck and cardiac abnormalities (coarctation of the aorta, bicuspid aortic valve).

148.

A. **True.** And 75 per cent of women presenting are aged over 50 years.

B. **True.** Few women with endometrial carcinoma are aged less than 40 years. However, 20–25 per cent of cases occur in premenopausal patients.

C. **True.**

D. **False.** Patients with ovarian dysgenesis require long-term oestrogen therapy; therefore a combined preparation is recommended. Endometrial cancer is rare in such patients.

E. **True.**

149.

A. **True.** About 30 per cent of deaths from pulmonary embolism occur antenatally, so it is important to diagnose the condition.

B. **False.** Venography and isotope lung scan can be used safely during pregnancy.

C. **True.** Side effect of heparin.

Thromboembolic disease

The most recent Confidential Enquiry into Maternal Deaths lists thrombosis and thromboembolism as the major direct cause of maternal death (33 per cent of all direct deaths), followed by hypertensive disease of pregnancy, sepsis, amniotic fluid embolism, haemorrhage, anaesthesia and cardiac disease. (*Why Mothers Die*)

150.

A. **True.** The onset is more common in someone who has had children, especially after the first child.

B. **True.** The nature of the symptoms is not as important as their premenstrual, cyclical nature causing disruption to life and improving when menstruation starts.

151.

A. **True.** The anterior shoulder becomes impacted against the symphysis pubis, and further descent of the fetus is prevented.

B. **False.** This problem occurs in 0.3–1.0 per cent of deliveries less than 4 kg birthweight, and in 3–7 per cent of deliveries of 4–4.5 kg birthweight.

C. **False.** The overall incidence of shoulder dystocia is 2 per cent, and almost half of the cases involve babies weighing less than 4 kg.

D. **False.** The manoeuvre involves marked flexion and abduction of the maternal hips.

E. **False.** These are commonly due to excessive neck traction. Of the brachial plexus injuries, Erb's palsy is the most common.

F. **False.** Episiotomy and McRobert's manoeuvre facilitate delivery of 50–60 per cent of cases.

G. **True.** For such infants, the rate of shoulder dystocia is 3–7 per cent in infants weighing more than 4 kg.

H. **True.** Even when controlled for other factors. Careful evaluation of such fetuses is recommended late in pregnancy, before vaginal delivery is attempted.

Other definitions of shoulder dystocia include:

- difficulty delivering the shoulder with the contraction subsequent to that which delivered the head;
- prolonged head-to-body delivery interval; and
- grades of severity based upon the interventions required.

152.

A. **False.** The puerperium describes the first 6 weeks after delivery. It is traditionally considered to be a period of rapid return to normal health, although recent studies show that many women experience significant health problems during this time.

B. **True.** A recent survey in a Birmingham hospital showed that 47 per cent reported at least one of a list of 25 different symptoms starting within 3 months of the birth and lasting for more than 6 weeks. All of these symptoms were new ones, and most continued for long periods of time. Two-thirds were unresolved at the time of enquiry 1–9 years after the birth.

C. **False.** The lochia usually clears completely within 4 weeks of delivery and consists of blood, leukocytes, shreds of decidua and organisms.

D. **True.** 10–14 days later after delivery the fundus will have disappeared behind the symphysis pubis and should not be palpable abdominally.

E. **True.** The effect of fatigue on the mother in the postnatal period is such that routine screening for postnatal anaemia is advocated in almost all centres.

F. **False.** 10–15 percent of women experience postnatal depression, and this may arise at any time within the first year after delivery.

153.

A. **True.** Primary amenorrhoea in the presence of breast development and in the absence of a uterus is seen in testicular feminization. The genotype is XY, but androgenic induction of the Wolffian system does not occur and as Mullerian inhibiting factor is still present the Mullerian system does not develop either. Thus, there is breast development without axillary or pubic hair.

B. **True.**

C. **True.**

Feminizing testes

An XY genotype may be associated with a female phenotype if there is:

- a failure of testicular development;
- enzymatic error in testosterone biosynthesis; or
- androgen insensitivity at the target organs, commonly known as testicular feminization.

154.

A. **False.** The incidence after normal pregnancy is 1:40–50 000.

B. **True.** And are usually aggressive tumours requiring chemotherapy.

C. **True.** This figure is approximate as there is usually no clinical indication to obtain further pathology.

D. **True.** Particularly if they have chest symptoms, since tumours occurring after a term delivery are commonly aggressive.

E. **True.** However, it is important to confirm that beta-hCG (human chorionic gonadotrophin) returns to normal after each subsequent pregnancy.

Trophoblastic disease

Poor prognostic indicators if:

- the antecedent pregnancy is a term delivery;
- the interval from the antecedent pregnancy is >12 months;
- the initial hCG concentration is >10^5 IU/L;
- there are multiple pulmonary metastases;
- there are metastases in brain and liver; and
- there is failure of prior chemotherapy with two or more drugs.

155.
A. **False.** It is an antagonist. It stimulates the synthesis of prostaglandins by the decidua, and causes uterine contractions.
B. **False.** Early referral is necessary, as it is not licensed for use after 7 weeks' gestation or 9 weeks' amenorrhoea.
C. **True.** Approximately 24–48 h after administration of mifepristone, the woman is admitted for application of a prostaglandin E_1 (PGE_1) vaginal pessary. 3 per cent will abort before readmission, 90 per cent within 6 h, and 99 per cent within 24 h of prostaglandin administration. The amount of bleeding is about three times more than a normal period, and lasts for 8 days on average. Follow-up is essential.

156.
A. **True.**
B. **True.**
C. **True.**
D. **True.**
E. **True.**

157.
A. **False.** Prolactin levels during lactation are dependent upon the strength, frequency and duration of suckling stimuli; basal prolactin levels are highest in the immediate puerperium, and decline slowly as suckling declines in later lactation. Reversion to non-pregnant levels occurs immediately after weaning.
B. **True.** Prolactin acts directly on the secretory cells of the breast to stimulate the synthesis of the milk proteins, e.g. casein.
C. **False.** The reverse is **True.** The relevant values are 7 mmol/L and 22 mmol/L.

158.

A. **False.** The oestrogenic actions include the stimulation of progesterone receptor status.

B. **True.**

C. **False.** The decrease in antithrombin III observed with tamoxifen is still within the normal range, and clinical trials have indicated no significant increase in thrombotic events.

D. **False.** This has been seen in rats, but this effect is unlikely to be a clinical problem at the doses currently used.

E. **False.** There have been many reports of a rapid and symptomatic growth of endometriosis.

159.

A. **False.** The relationship between gestational age and risk of complications is inverse, i.e. as one increases, the other decreases.

B. **True.**

C. **False.** In cases of PROM less than 28 weeks, the survival rate is more than 60 per cent because the time between PROM and the onset of labour is, on average, 4 weeks. After 26 weeks, fetal lung maturation can be induced with corticosteroids.

D. **False.** The risk of amnionitis is increased if vaginal examinations are performed; however, sometimes it may be necessary in order to determine cervical conditions.

E. **False.** Unless specific culture results are known, the antibiotics usually recommended in PROM are ampicillin 1–2 g intravenously every 4–6 h, plus netilimicin. If the mother is allergic to penicillin, erythromycin can be used. Cardiotocography is mandatory to monitor fetal well-being, and the biophysical profile is recommended. Other procedures such as serial monitoring of the white cell count, the level of C-reactive protein, and temperature are also used to screen for infection.

F. **True.** Compared with 6.5 per cent of patients delivered by elective Caesarean section at term, 10–25 per cent after labour at term, and 35–59 per cent after preterm labour.

160.

A. **True.** Urethral caruncle is of unknown cause, but may be associated with chronic *Trichomonas* infection. It is commonly seen in postmenopausal women and can recur after surgical treatment.

B. **False.** Usually asymptomatic, it may cause pain, bleeding and dysuria.

C. **True.** Excision biopsy followed by local or systemic oestrogen.

D. **False.** It is usually found on the posterior aspect of the external meatus.

E. **False.** Urethral caruncle is a benign red polyp or lesion covered by transitional epithelial.

161.

A. **False.** The most common problem after delivery is tiredness, affecting 54 per cent after the first 2 months. This may become a chronic problem; 12 per cent of women report extreme exhaustion arising as a new symptom and persisting for at least 6 weeks.

B. **False.** They are rarely encountered before the 14th day of the postnatal period.

C. **False.** Mother should allow baby to continue to feed as normal.

162.

A. **True.** Thrombosis and thromboembolism were responsible for the highest proportion (23 per cent) of direct maternal deaths recorded in a recent report (*Why Mothers Die*, 2001). 48 per cent occurred postpartum, and 69 per cent followed Caesarean section.

B. **True.** Other risk factors include previous thromboembolism, obesity, immobilization, and operative delivery. In two-thirds of cases, death occurred after the 7th day of the postnatal period.

Risk factors for venous thromboembolism in pregnancy

General:

Age over 35 years; immobility; obesity; operative delivery; pre-eclampsia; parity greater than four; surgical procedure in pregnancy or puerperium, e.g. postpartum sterilization; previous deep venous thrombosis (DVT); excessive blood loss; paraplegia; sickle-cell disease; inflammatory bowel disease and urinary tract infection; dehydration and thrombophilia.

Congenital:

Antithrombin deficiency; protein C deficiency; protein S deficiency; factor V Leiden; prothrombin gene variant.

Acquired:

Lupus anticoagulant; anticardiolipin antibodies.

163.

A. **False.** However, episiotomy is recommended in cases of forceps delivery or where a tear is thought to be inevitable.

B. **False.** This problem more often complicates midline (median) episiotomies.

C. **False.** There is no evidence to support this.

Episiotomy

The tissues incised by an episiotomy are:

- skin and subcutaneous tissues;
- vaginal mucosa;
- the urogenital septum (mostly fascia, but also the transverse perineal muscle);
- intercolumnar fascia or the superior fascia of pelvic diaphragm; and
- the lowermost fibres of the puborectalis portions of the levator ani muscle (if the episiotomy is mediolateral and deep).

164.
A. **True.**
B. **True.** The majority of whom remain symptomatic at 5 years.
C. **True.** In such instances, up to 40 per cent of women suffer early voiding difficulties. Late voiding difficulties occur in up to 20 per cent of women after colposuspension. Intermittent self-catheterization should be taught beforehand.
D. **False.** Cure rates are unaffected.

Conservative management of urinary incontinence includes:

- Exercise/re-education
- Pelvic floor exercises
- Vaginal cones/perineometer
- Bladder drill
- Biofeedback
- Electrical stimulation
- Medication
- Phenylpropanolamine
- Oestrogen replacement therapy
- Devices
- Tampon
- Femassist (an occlusive device which sits over the urethral orifice)
- Continence guard (intravaginal device)

165.
A. **False.** The definition does not differ with severity of disease, i.e. whether insulin is required or not.
B. **False.** In GDM the HbA1c is normal, whereas in overt DM it is elevated.
C. **False.** As GDM usually develops late, organogenesis is usually complete.

Haemoglobin A1 (HbA1)

Glucose influences the slow glycosylation of haemoglobin during the life cycle of the red cell, so that a high HbA1 level reflects a high average plasma glucose concentration. In non-diabetics the level is about 5 per cent, but may be as high as 20 per cent in newly diagnosed diabetics.

In normal subjects the HbA1 level averages 6 per cent throughout pregnancy. It is raised in diabetics, and although it falls as pregnancy advances, it is always higher than normal. In diabetic pregnancy the level should be as near to 6 per cent as possible, and values above 10 per cent should be viewed with concern.

166.

A. **False.** 46XX. Women with molar pregnancies have a high incidence of balanced translocations (incidence 0.5 to 2.5 per 1000 pregnancies). Risk is also increased in teenagers and in women aged over 35 years. The risk of recurrence of molar pregnancy in a woman with a history of the same is increased 20-fold. While other factors such as diet and blood group have been suggested, the evidence for these is weak. (*Dewhurst's Textbook of Obstetrics and Gynaecology for Postgraduates*, 6th edn)

B. **True.** Complete mole arises from the fertilization of an empty ovum, i.e. one where the nucleus is either absent or non-functional. The sperm duplicates its own chromosomes.

C. **False.**

D. **False.** It is triploid, again paternally derived. The fetus usually survives to 8–9 weeks.

E. **False.** The fetus rarely survives to term, often with multiple anomalies.

167.

A. **False.** Thalamocortical connections do not develop until after 22 weeks, so the fetus will not feel pain before this period.

B. **True.** But it is unlikely that there is fetal awareness until 26 weeks' gestation.

168.

A. **False.** Some claim that biofeedback and hypnotherapy have lower success rate, but bladder drill has been successfully used to treat idiopathic detrusor instability.

B. **True.** Urinalysis and mid-stream urine (MSU) are essential. Cystourethroscopy is indicated, and those with normal findings are often improved by bladder distension and urethral dilatation.

C. **True.**

169.

A. **False.** This describes a fourth-degree tear. A third-degree tear describes extension into the rectal sphincter.

B. **False.** Second-degree tears involve the perineal muscles and skin only.

C. **False.** These tears involve disruption of the fibres of the external and internal anal sphincters and mucosa.

Perineum

The perineum is bounded by the levatores ani above, by the vulva and anus below, and by the pelvic outlet (subpubic angle, ischiopubic rami, ischial tuberosities, sacrotuberous ligaments and coccyx) laterally. It is divided into a urogenital triangle anteriorly and an anal triangle posteriorly. There is a superficial fascia of fat and a deeper membranous fascia (the fascia Colles), which extends over the pubis as the fascia of scar.

170.

A. **False.** 2 per cent.

B. **True.** This narrows the lower segment, resulting in a falsely low-lying placenta.

C. **False.** The diagnostic accuracy is similar to that of the transabdominal route, but the false-positive and -negative rates are lower, helping to prevent unnecessary admissions to hospital

D. **True.** This is traditionally the modality of diagnosis of placenta praevia. Difficulties with imaging can arise in an obese woman, or when the fetal head or maternal symphysis pubis obscures the posteriorly implanted placenta.

E. **True.** Numerous prospective observational trials have used TVS to diagnose placenta praevia. None has experienced any haemorrhagic complication. TAS in the second trimester is associated with a high false-positive rate, and TVS will reclassify 26–60 per cent of cases. Benefits of using TVS include reduced scanning time and superior views, particularly of placentas situated posteriorly.

Transvaginal ultrasound

Advantages:

- Avoids the need for a full bladder. A partially filled bladder helps with orientation.
- No problem with acoustic shadowing from the symphysis pubis or the fetal head.
- Fewer problems with attenuation of sound waves from the obese patient.
- Generally a comfortable procedure.
- The procedure time is shortened.

Disadvantages:

- It is an 'invasive' procedure and may not be acceptable to some patients.
- There is a theoretical risk of provoking haemorrhage form a low-lying placenta.
- Possibility of introducing infection when the membranes are ruptured.

171.

A. **False.** Pulmonary thromboembolism (PTE) is a major cause of maternal mortality. Clinical diagnosis is unreliable, and up to 70 per cent of those who suffer a fatal PTE may exhibit no previous signs of deep venous thrombosis (DVT) or PTE. In order to reduce the mortality and morbidity associated with PTE, the identification of those at risk and provision of appropriate thromboprophylaxis is essential.

B. **True.** While pregnancy and the puerperium are themselves important risk factors, age, high parity, obesity and Caesarean section are also significant.

C. **False.** A previous history of thromboembolism has, until recently, been considered an indication for long-term anticoagulation during pregnancy. Prospective studies suggest, however, that the risk of recurrence during pregnancy in patients with a history of a single episode of thromboembolism, not receiving prophylaxis is only 1–5 per cent. Taking into account the potential hazards of anticoagulation in pregnancy, the need for prophylactic therapy in women with a single episode of DVT in the past with no additional risk factors has been questioned.

D. **False.** All women who undergo emergency Caesarean section are at moderate risk, and in need of prophylaxis, normally in the form of unfractionated heparin. Thromboembolic deterrent stockings are also advised if the patient is deemed to be in the high-risk category.

E. **False.** These patients are deemed low risk, and as such early mobilization and adequate hydration are sufficient.

F. **True.** High-risk patients include those undergoing extended major pelvic surgery (e.g. Caesarean hysterectomy), patients with a personal or family history of DVT, pulmonary embolism or thrombophilia, paralysis of lower limbs and patients with antiphospholipid antibody.

Thrombosis and thromboembolism

These are the major direct causes of maternal death, with a rate of 16.5 per million maternities. They account for 33 per cent of all direct maternal deaths. While the rate of deaths due to thromboembolic disease in pregnancy has fallen (21.8 per million maternities in a previous Confidential Enquiry into Maternal Deaths), the number of deaths due to thromboembolic disease in other women has risen. (*Why Mothers Die*)

172.

A. **True.**

B. **True.** Full anticoagulation with heparin and warfarin is a clear contraindication to spinal or epidural anaesthesia because of the risk of spinal haematoma. The situation regarding low-dose heparin and low molecular-weight heparin used for prophylaxis is more controversial. Guidelines for anaesthetists have suggested delaying the siting of a block until 4–6 h after the last low-dose heparin injection.

C. **False.** Side effects of heparin include osteoporosis, which may result in fractures in around 2.2 per cent of women receiving prolonged antenatal low-dose heparin therapy. Thrombocytopenia is also recognized, and the platelet count should therefore be checked regularly.

D. **False.** If low-dose unfractionated heparin is employed, the normal dose is 5000 IU b.i.d. Treatment should continue until the patient is fully mobile. Warfarin can safely be substituted for heparin 1 week after delivery. At this time the risk of secondary postpartum haemorrhage is reduced, and breast-feeding can be safely continued.

173.

A. **True.** The short-term increase in the risk of breast cancer after full term delivery is maximal 3–4 years after delivery.

B. **False.** The worse prognosis for women developing breast cancer soon after pregnancy is exaggerated further in those aged less than 30 years.

C. **True.** As well as greater tumour size, there is a greater risk of metastatic disease.

D. **False.** The correct figure is 7 per cent.

E. **False.** Studies show this to be between 56 and 70 per cent.

F. **False.** Recommendations are for a delay of 2 years.

G. **False.** There is no evidence to support this.

H. **True.** There is no evidence to support termination of pregnancy as a beneficial treatment option in this regard.

174.

A. **True.** For example, systemic lupus erythematosus, autoimmune thrombocytopenia, rheumatoid arthritis.

B. **True.** These are the two antiphospholipid antibodies, which are recognized as clinically important.

C. **False.** The rate of pregnancy loss in the presence of anticardiolipin antibody and lupus anticoagulant may be as high as 90 per cent.

D. **False.** The correct figure is 5 per cent.

E. **False.** The term is a misnomer. Lupus anticoagulant increases the tendency to clot.

F. **True.** However, the proportion of patients with anticardiolipin antibodies with lupus anticoagulant is smaller.

G. **False.** Clinical criteria for the diagnosis include: autoimmune thrombocytopenia, recurrent pregnancy loss, arterial or venous thrombosis. Laboratory criteria include: lupus anticoagulant, moderate to high levels of IgG anticardiolipin antibodies.

H. **True.** Other therapies used include prednisolone, immunoglobulin and heparin.

175.

A. **True.** Malpresentation, placenta accreta but (not praevia) and necrobiosis are recognized complications.

B. **True.**

C. **False.**

D. **True.**

Complication of fibroids during pregnancy:

- Fibroids may enlarge and soften during pregnancy.

- Infarction of pedunculated fibroids is more common and manifests as subacute abdominal pain which may be associated with peritoneal irritation and guarding. It may be difficult to distinguish infarction from acute appendicitis and pyelonephritis.

- Conservative treatment, i.e. bed rest and analgesia, usually results in symptom improvement in approximately 10 days.

- Torsion of a pedunculated fibroid occurs more commonly in the puerperal period as uterine involution and lax abdominal wall muscles allow greater mobility of abdominal contents.

Clinical signs are in keeping with an acute abdomen, although guarding and rigidity are usually absent.

Differential diagnosis includes accident to ovarian cyst, intestinal volvulus, appendicitis, ureteric colic and rectus sheath haematoma. It may be necessary to remove the fibroid in question. (*Dewhurst's Textbook of Obstetrics and Gynaecology for Postgraduates, 6th edn*)

176.

A. **True.** Also there is increase incidence of spontaneous abortion.

B. **False.** Due to sickling crisis, when red blood cells clump together.

C. **False.** The risk is 1:4. The carrier rate in the UK is 1:10 000.

Haematological disorders

Features of sickle-cell trait in pregnancy:

- Women with sickle-cell trait (8.5 per cent of black women) have a normal haematocrit but, under certain circumstances such as physical stress, dehydration and hypoxia, sickling and resultant thrombosis may occur. This in turn may result in infarction of small renal vessels and cause parenchymal infarction.

- Thalassaemias are due to defective synthesis of globin chains, leading to an imbalance and precipitation of these chains within the red cell precursors. Precipitation of these chains in mature red cells leads to haemolysis.

Beta-thalassaemia:

In the homozygous state, normal beta chain production is either absent or very reduced. This produces an excess of alpha chains, which results in increased quantities of other forms of haemoglobin. Further subdivision is into thalassaemia major (severe anaemia requiring regular transfusions), thalassaemia intermedia (rarely requiring transfusions) and thalassaemia minor or trait, which is the symptomless heterozygous state.

Alpha-thalassaemia:

This is due to deletion of one or both genes on each chromosome 16. If all four genes are absent, no alpha chains are present and Hb Barts is present – this form of haemoglobin cannot carry oxygen and therefore is not compatible with life and results in death *in utero* or soon after delivery.

If three genes are deleted, Hb H disease is said to exist. Patients are not usually transfusion dependent. If one or two genes are deleted, this is called alpha-thalassaemia trait and manifests clinically as microcytosis without anaemia.

177.
A. **True.** It is postulated that this is the common mechanism by which aspirin might work in the prophylaxis of pre-eclampsia, the management of primary antiphospholipid syndrome (PAPS) and thromboprophylaxis.
B. **False.** There was only a 12 per cent reduction, which was not significant.
C. **True.** Subgroup analysis of the CLASP trial (see References) suggested this. Early-onset PET is more severe. Risk factors for early-onset PET are hypertension requiring treatment before pregnancy, renal disease and past history of early-onset PET in a previous pregnancy.

178.

A. **False.** They originate from smooth muscle, but also have a connective tissue component.
B. **False.** The incidence is highest in the fifth decade.
C. **False.** There is no evidence to support this. Fibroids do appear to be sensitive to oestrogen however, in that they grow in the childbearing period and regress in the menopausal period.
D. **True.** Other types include subserosal, intramural and cervical.
E. **False.** Less than 1 per cent of all fibroids are malignant; they are called leiomyosarcomas.
F. **True.** Direct extension via the venous system as far as the right side of the heart has been described.
G. **False.** They may arise from the smooth muscle of erectile structures.
H. **False.** Subserous fibroids project from the peritoneal surface of the uterus. Submucous fibroids project into the uterine cavity.
I. **True.** Thus, subserous fibroids are more likely than submucous fibroids to change in this way.
J. **False.** They should be left undisturbed due to the risk of haemorrhage.
K. **False.** Rupture of the myomectomy scar is rare. Vaginal delivery may well be possible.
L. **True.**

Radiological embolization

The procedure is performed by an interventional radiologist under fluoroscopic guidance. A catheter is introduced through the femoral vasculature into the main arteries that supply the uterus. Microscopic particles called polyvinyl alcohol (PVA) are injected through the catheter to occlude the blood vessels supplying the fibroid. During the process, the radiologist injects contrast dye in order to visualize the vessels. After the process, catheters are removed and direct pressure is applied to the puncture site. The patient would be required to lie flat for 5–6 h post procedure in order to ensure minimal bleeding.

179.

A. **True.** A clinical feature of mitral stenosis.
B. **True.**
C. **True.** Early diastolic murmur indicates full evaluation of cardiac status to role out any cardiac lesion.

Complications of mitral stenosis in pregnancy

Mitral stenosis remains the most potentially lethal pre-existing heart condition in pregnancy. It may be missed during the routine antenatal examination because the murmur is diastolic. Clinically, tachycardia is a response to failure to increase stroke volume. This results in a decreased time for emptying of the left atrium, which further accelerates the tachycardia, and thus a vicious circle is formed. Pulmonary oedema is precipitated, provoking anxiety and exacerbating the tachycardia. Options for treatment are balloon valvotomy when the clinical condition has improved, or beta-blocking drugs if the mitral valve is unsuitable for such repair. Epidural analgesia is recommended for labour as long as the mitral stenosis is not complicated by pulmonary hypertension.

180.
A. **True.** There is three-fold increase in the rate of placental abruption compared with normal pregnant women.
B. **False.** 5 mg folic acid.
C. **False.** 1:80 is the usual incidence of epilepsy.
D. **True.**
E. **True.** Carbamazepine, phenobarbitone and phenytoin are associated with neonatal bleeding, and vitamin K is recommended for the mother before delivery and for the neonate after delivery.
F. **False.** Epilepsy shows no consistent relationship with pregnancy, but rheumatoid arthritis and migraine tend to improve.

Epilepsy and pregnancy

Increased maternal plasma volume, delayed gastro-intestinal absorption and increased hepatic clearance can result in subtherapeutic levels of medication. Vaginal bleeding is thought to be more common, probably due to anticonvulsant-induced vitamin K deficiency.

Fetal complications of epilepsy:

- The fetus is thought to be extremely tolerant of grand mal seizures, and the transient hypoxia inherent does not seem to cause any long-term harm. Following a seizure, fetal bradycardia is common and may persist for up to 20 min.
- The risk of congenital abnormalities is two to three times that of the general population.
- The risk of birth defect increases with the number of anticonvulsants used.
- The most common defects are cleft lip and palate, neural tube defects and craniofacial dysmorphism. Pathogenesis is thought to be multifactorial.

181.

A. **True.**

B. **True.**

C. **False.** A frequency of 40 Hz is best for fast fibres, and a frequency of 10 Hz is best for slow fibres. Fast fibres are needed to control genuine stress incontinence, while slow fibres are those used to control detrusor instability.

D. **True.** Conservative management should be the first approach for the majority of women.

182.

A. **False.** 3–5 per cent of ovarian germ cell tumours are malignant. Most germ cell tumours occur in children and adolescents.

B. **True.** However, cystic teratomas or dermoids are the most common germ cell tumour overall.

C. **True.** These tumours commonly arise in dysgenetic ovaries, and thus preconceptual genetic counselling may be advisable.

D. **True.** Other biochemical tumour markers include alpha-fetoprotein and Ca125.

E. **False.** These tumours are overtly bilateral in only 10–15 per cent of cases, and covertly bilateral in 15 per cent of cases.

Ovarian germ cell tumours

Survival rates for primary ovarian carcinoma:

- Stage Ia = 85 per cent.
- Stage Ib–IIa = 40 per cent.
- Stage IIb = 25 per cent.
- Stage IIc–III = 15 per cent.
- Stage VI = <5 per cent.

Dysgerminomas:

- Occur in both sexes (dysgerminoma of the ovary is identical with the seminoma of the testis).
- Unlike most other ovarian tumours, they are often chromatin-negative.
- Bilateral in one-third of cases.
- Macroscopically, the tumour is solid except for any degenerative cystic changes.
- Microscopically, it is composed of large cell arranged in bundles or alevoli separated by a characteristic network of connective tissue which is infiltrated with lymphocytes. The appearances mimic those of the gonad at a very early stage of its development, and the large tumour cells resemble primitive ova.
- Most dysgerminomas are malignant.

183.

A. **True.**

B. **True.**

C. **True.**

D. **True.**

E. **False.** Genetic analysis suggests a single recessive trait.

F. **False.** More common in dizygotic twins.

G. **False.** Magnesium sulphate is the drug of choice in parts of the world where eclampsia is common. It is also becoming more popular in the UK.

H. **True.** Blindness may be due to central arterial and venous thrombosis, retinal oedema and detachment. Pre-eclampsia can also cause liver failure (a late manifestation), micro-angiopathic haemolysis, thrombocytopenia and low cardiac output.

Magnesium sulphate treatment of pre-eclampsia

Eclampsia should be treated with intravenous magnesium sulphate, followed by a magnesium sulphate infusion to prevent further seizures.

Loading dose:

- 4 g (8 mL) $MgSO_4$ 50% diluted in 20 mL of 0.9% sodium chloride, given i.v. over 5–10 min.
- Repeat 2–4 g i.v. if seizures continue.

Maintenance dose:

1 g $MgSO_4$ per hour. Add 25 g (i.e. 50 mL of 50% $MgSO_4$) to 250 mL of 0.9% NaCl and infuse at a rate of 12 mL/h.

Therapeutic range: 2–4 mmol/L (4.0–8.0 mg/dL).

Dose alterations:

- Oliguria (≤100 mL over 4 h) or urea >10 mmol/L: give 1 g/h maintenance dose and measure Mg levels more frequently.
- ALT >250 IU/L: measure Mg levels every 2–4 h.
- Mg level >4 mmol/L: decrease maintenance dose to 0.5 or 1 g/h, depending on level.
- Mg level <1.7 mmol/L: consider further 2-g i.v. bolus over 20 min. Increase maintenance dose to 2.5 g/h.
- Mg level 1.7–2.0 mmol/L: although this is strictly 'subtherapeutic', provided that the patient is stable and levels are not persistently <1.7 mmol/L, it is reasonable to continue with a 2 g/h maintenance dose.

Toxicity:

- Loss of patellar reflex, weakness.
- Nausea, feeling of warmth, flushing, weakness.
- Somnolence, double vision, slurred speech   Mg level 5 mmol/L.
- Muscle paralysis, respiratory arrest   Mg level 6.0–7.5 mmol/L.
- Cardiac arrest   Mg level >12 mmol/L.

184.

A. **False.** The correct figure is 85 per cent, and of these 60–70 per cent will require suturing.

B. **False.** This is all true apart from bladder.

C. **False.** As might be expected, the problem is thought to be caused by nerve damage and direct trauma.

Classification of perineal tears:

- First degree: involving skin only.
- Second degree: injury to the perineum involving perineal muscles but not involving the anal sphincter.
- Third degree: injury to the perineum involving the anal sphincter complex (external anal sphincter (EAS) and internal anal sphincter (IAS)).
  - 3a: <50 per cent of the EAS thickness torn.
  - 3b: >50 per cent of the EAS thickness torn.
  - 3c: IAS torn.
- Fourth degree: injury to the perineum involving the anal sphincter complex (EAS and IAS) and mucosa.

185.

A. **False.** If hCG levels reach the normal range (serum 0–4 IU/L, urine 0–24 IU/L) within 56 days of evacuation, follow-up will be limited to 6 months. Patients requiring short follow-up can start a new pregnancy immediately. All other patients require 2-year follow-up. It is reasonable to allow a further pregnancy once hCG has been normal for 6 months. In this group the risk of choriocarcinoma developing is 1:286.

B. **False.**

C. **True.**

D. **True.**

E. **False.**

186.

A. **True.**

B. **True.** The most recent study estimates it to be 0.96 per cent for low-dose pill users, and 0.5 per cent for non-users.

C. **False.** There is no evidence of an association of HRT with venous thromboembolism. HRT need not be stopped prior to surgery.

187.
A. **False.** The score should be lower than 2. Otherwise, the World Federation for Ultrasound in Medicine and Biology (WFUMB) warns that to operate with TIS >4 for more than 5 min is potentially hazardous.
B. **True.**
C. **True.** Modern machines usually allow the operator to select an optimum frequency. High-frequency ultrasound provides better resolution at the expense of penetration.
D. **False.**

188.
A. **True.** The number of women who experience BTB is considerable and it is a difficult management problem.
B. **True.**
C. **True.** It originates from an endometrium dominated by progestational influence; hence the endometrium is atrophic and yields little to the biopsy instrument.
D. **True.**
E. **False.** The BTB rate is not much better with a higher dose of progestin (5 mg MPA) compared with the lower dose (2.5 mg).

HRT – side effects

Gastro-intestinal problems and bloating, weight changes, breast enlargement and tenderness, premenstrual-like syndrome, sodium and fluid retention, changes in liver function, cholestatic jaundice, altered blood lipids, rashes and chloasma, changes in libido, depression, headache, migraine, dizziness, leg cramps, contact lenses may irritate, transdermal delivery systems may cause contact sensitization, nasal spray may cause local irritation, rhinorrhoea and epistaxis.

189.
A. **True.** At least 20 per cent of women suffer from stress incontinence for 3 months after delivery, and three-quarters of them will still be incontinent a year later, without treatment.
B. **False.** 20 per cent, and 75 per cent of them will still be incontinent a year later, without treatment
C. **False.** Postnatal exercises are not effective in its prevention, although they do appear to reduce the incidence of other problems such as perineal pain and depression.
D. **True.**

190.
A. **True.** The miscarriage rate is estimated at 15–20 per cent overall, and may be even higher as many pregnancies are thought to miscarry before they are clinically apparent.
B. **False.** hCG levels double every 48 h in a normal pregnancy.
C. **False.** It may take 1–2 weeks to fall to this level.
D. **True.** In a healthy pregnancy in a normal anatomical location, the beta hCG level will double within 2 days.
E. **True.** Nor does hCG.

191.

A. True.

B. False.

C. True.

D. True.

192.

A. True.   Meta-analysis of trials of oxytocics in the third stage suggests that their routine use decreases postpartum maternal blood loss by 30–40 per cent, decreases the need for blood transfusions, and improves Hb levels.

B. False.   It should be avoided in hypertensive patients.

C. False.   This clinical picture is a contraindication to the use of ergometrine and, at the very least, extreme caution and senior advice should be utilized.

D. True.

E. True.   It is postulated that waiting 60 rather than 30 min before resorting to manual removal for retained placenta will halve the number of women requiring an anaesthetic for this reason.

Management of labour

For routine management of the third stage of labour ergometrine 500 micrograms with oxytocin 5 units (Syntometrine 1 mL) is given by intramuscular injection on delivery of the anterior shoulder or, at the latest, immediately after the baby is delivered. If ergometrine is inappropriate (e.g. in pre-eclampsia), oxytocin alone may be given by intramuscular injection (unlicensed use).

193.

A. True.   Neuromuscular electrical stimulation is widely used. A low-intensity, low-frequency stimulation has a 'trophic' effect on neuromuscular activity, i.e. it enhances blood supply, encourages muscle protein synthesis, and encourages axonal sprouting to improve re-innervation. Maximum intensity, low-frequency current is best for detrusor instability.

B. True.   Psychotherapy is bladder drill, which is effective in the short term.

C. True.

D. True.   S3 sacral nerve stimulation is a new form of neuromodulation, which has been effective in recent trials.

E. False.   Distigmine is used to treat urinary retention.

194.

A. False.   Endometrioid carcinomas occur in the majority of cases. Subtypes include typical (60 per cent), with squamous differentiation (25 per cent), secretory and ciliated.

B. True.

C. True.   Clear-cell adenocarcinoma occurs in 3–6 per cent of cases, and is the third most common cell type after endometrioid and serous papillary adenocarcinoma.

D. True.   But when present they are common in the cervix.

E. True.

195.

A. **True.** It is a weak anti-oestrogen that works at the hypothalamic level to initiate the changes needed to produce an ovulatory cycle.

B. **False.** It blocks oestrogen receptors in the hypothalamus, and interferes with the feedback mechanism, thus stimulating release of the gonadotrophins, FSH and LH, to initiate the changes needed to produce an ovulatory cycle.

C. **True.** Rarely more than twins. Other side effects are hot flushes, mood swings, ovarian cysts and, rarely, visual disturbances.

D. **True.** If testosterone level has been elevated, dexamethasone 0.5 mg/day may be given in the follicular phase of the cycle up to the time of ovulation.

E. **True.** Decreased amplitude and frequency of GnRH secretion are associated with excess exercise, stress and weight loss (hypogonadotrophic hypo-oestrogenism).

F. **False.** Failure of ovarian response occurs in resistant ovary syndrome, premature ovarian failure and gonadal dysgenesis.

G. **True.** It works better when the gonadotrophin levels are normal. In hypogonadotrophic hypo-oestrogenism induction of ovulation is more difficult.

H. **False.** This used to be the case. However, medical therapy is now recommended as first-line treatment.

I. **True.** The success rate for treatment of ovarian disorders is as much as 80–90 per cent compared with 30 per cent for other causes of infertility.

Anti-oestrogens (clomiphene and tamoxifen)

These are used for the treatment of female infertility due to oligomenorrhoea or secondary amenorrhoea. They induce gonadotrophin release by occupying oestrogen receptors in the hypothalamus, thereby interfering with feedback mechanisms.

Clomiphene citrate:

This should not normally be used for longer than six cycles.

Contraindications: hepatic disease, ovarian cysts, hormone-dependent tumours or abnormal uterine bleeding of undetermined cause, pregnancy.

Side effects: visual disturbance, ovarian hyperstimulation, hot flushes, abdominal discomfort, occasionally nausea, vomiting, depression, insomnia, breast tenderness, headache, intermenstrual spotting, menorrhagia, endometriosis, convulsions, weight gain, rash, dizziness, hair loss.

Dose: 50 mg daily for 5 days, starting within about 5 days of onset of menstruation (preferably on 2nd day). Second course of 100 mg daily for 5 days in the absence of ovulation.

196.
A. **True.** Perineal massage practised antenatally has been shown to reduce perineal trauma at delivery and later dyspareunia. Perineal massage during the second stage of labour – otherwise known as 'ironing out' the perineum – does not do any harm. Yet in a randomized controlled trial in Australia, it did not prevent perineal trauma, later dyspareunia or urinary incontinence.
B. **False.**
C. **False.**
D. **False.**
E. **False.**

197.
A. **True.** There have been occasional reports of gynaecomastia and erectile dysfunction.
B. **False.** Most often erectile dysfunction is due to psychological factors but there may be vascular, neurogenic or endocrine abnormalities.
C. **True.**
D. **True.**
E. **False.** Peyronie's disease causes an angulation of the penis, and sildenafil may lead to priapism.

Sildenafil (Viagra)

This is used to treat erectile dysfunction, and given by mouth.

Dose: initially 50 mg (elderly 25 mg) approximately 1 hour before sexual activity.

Side effects: dyspepsia, headache, flushing, dizziness, visual disturbances and increased intra-ocular pressure, nasal congestion, hypersensitivity reactions (including rash), priapism and painful, red eyes and serious cardiovascular events reported. Appropriate assessment should be carried out before prescribing sildenafil. Since sildenafil is administered systemically, it has a potential for drug interactions; it should not be used in those receiving nitrates.

198.
A. **False.** Smoking is a risk factor with contraceptive pill usage, regardless of age. However, COCP may be taken by smokers up until the age of 35 years.
B. **False.** Less than 5 per cent. The COCP is under-used in women in their 40s.
C. **False.** It contains 20–50 mg, i.e. 0.02–0.05 mg.
D. **True.** Inhibition of LH secretion is attributed to the progestogen.
E. **True.** Hydantoins and barbiturates potentiate hepatic conjugation and excretion.

Combined oral contraceptive pill (COCP)

Absolute contraindications:
Breast cancer, history of deep venous thrombosis (DVT) or thromboembolism, active liver disease (congenital/acquired), concurrent treatment with rifampicin, familial hyperlipidaemia, previous arterial thrombosis, pregnancy, undiagnosed abnormal vaginal bleeding.

Relative contraindications:
Smoking, age >35 years, obesity, breast-feeding.

Death due to the pill in those aged >35 years is eight times more common among women who smoke, and either the pill or the smoking should be stopped at this stage. Low-risk, non-smokers may continue the COCP until the menopause.

199.
A. **False.** It involves the lower two-thirds.
B. **True.** 38–73 per cent of patients complain of pruritis. Other symptoms are vulval pain/soreness and a lump/lesion.
C. **True.** 60 per cent of cases involve non-hairy skin exclusively.
D. **False.** The most common site is the posterior one-third, extending to the frenulum of the fourchette.
E. **False.** 33 per cent are unifocal, and 66 per cent are multifocal.

200.
A. **False.** Both CVS and amniocentesis may be employed after 10 weeks and 3 days when the fetus pole is more than 39 mm.
B. **False.** The miscarriage rate after CVS at 11–14 weeks is 2–3 per cent. The miscarriage risk for amniocentesis is 1–2 per cent.
C. **False.** In 1 per cent the mosaicism will be limited to the placenta, and does not affect the fetus.

201.
A. **True.** There are various classifications of female sexual dysfunction. The main causes are vaginismus, lack of libido, difficulty in reaching orgasm, vaginal dryness or soreness (often linked to infection or loss of oestrogen pre- or post-menopause).
B. **False.** Vaginismus is defined as the involuntary spasm of the muscle surrounding the vaginal outlet and lower third of the vagina.
C. **False.** Vaginismus occurs in response to an actual or imagined attempt at penetration.

Vaginismus

Vaginismus is the involuntary constriction or spasm of the muscles surrounding the vaginal outlet and lower one-third of the vagina. It occurs in women of any age, and the spectrum extends from unconsummated marriages to painful, but possible, intercourse. Although vaginismus may make a woman fearful of sexual activity and limit her overall responsiveness, more commonly she experiences little problem with sexual arousal. Vaginal lubrication occurs normally, non-coital activity can be pleasurable, and the orgasmic response is often intact.

202.

A. **False.** Vulval atrophy is a normal finding in elderly women and is often asymptomatic. Thus, it does not always need treatment.

B. **False.** Vulval dystrophy is not an indication for such aggressive surgery.

C. **True.**

D. **False.** Squamous cell hyperplasia replaces hyperplastic dystrophy.

E. **True.** As is melanoma in-situ.

F. **True.** It is not evidence of a distinct dermatological condition. These cases are classified as lichen sclerosis with associated squamous cell hyperplasia. When VIN occurs with dystrophy, both diagnoses should be reported.

G. **False.** It is often worse at night, and can cause insomnia if severe.

H. **True.** A thorough systemic review is essential, as a vulval dermatosis may be part of a generalized dermatological condition, e.g. lichen planus, eczema, psoriasis, vitiligo and allergic dermatitis.

I. **True.** As can Behçet's disease, Crohn's disease, ulcerative colitis and amyloidosis.

Classification of vulval disorders (ISSVD 1989):

- Non-neoplastic disorders of the vulva.
- Squamous cell hyperplasia (formerly hyperplastic dystrophy).
- Lichen sclerosis (formerly hypoplastic dystrophy).
- Other dermatoses
- Vulval intraepithelial neoplasia (VIN).
- Squamous VIN.
  - VIN I: Mild dysplasia.
  - VIN II: Moderate dysplasia.
  - VIN III: Severe dysplasia with carcinoma in-situ.
- Non-squamous VIN.
  - Paget's disease.
  - Melanoma in-situ.

203.

A. **False.** However, fibroids may cause pain due to stretching of peritoneum, torsion or local pressure effects.

B. **True.** Similar reproducible trigger points may be found in the paracervical tissue.

C. **True.** Studies show that 48 per cent of women with chronic pelvic pain have such a history, compared with 6 per cent of the pain-free population.

204.

A. **True.** Whereas primary dysmenorrhoea commences at the onset of menses.

B. **False.** Mefanamic acid is beneficial for dysmenorrhoea due to its action as an inhibitor of prostaglandin synthesis. Tranexamic acid is an antifibrinolytic used to treat menorrhagia.

205.

A. **False.** Tamoxifen is very similar to clomiphene (in structure and actions), both being non-steroidal compounds. It is both an oestrogen agonist and antagonist.

B. **True.** *In vitro*, the oestrogen binding affinity for its receptor is 100- to 1000-fold greater than that of tamoxifen. Thus, tamoxifen must be present in a concentration 100- to 1000-fold greater than oestrogen in order to maintain inhibition of breast cancer cells.

C. **True.** In postmenopausal women, with low endogenous oestrogen levels, tamoxifen has a weak oestrogenic effect.

D. **True.** The benefit of tamoxifen is evident, no matter what the age of the patient or type of tumour.

E. **True.** There have been many reports of endometrial cancer occurring in women receiving tamoxifen treatment. Annual endometrial surveillance of postmenopausal women is recommended. If premenopausal women are ovulating, no further intervention is necessary.

206.

A. **True.**   HDN results from a lack of vitamin K, and infants present with systemic bleeding. The classical form occurs between 1 and 7 days after birth.

B. **True.**   Oral vitamin K is now recommended.

207.

A. **True.**

B. **True.**

C. **True.**

D. **False.**

E. **True.**

Ca125

Ca125 is elevated in 50 per cent of stage 1 and in 90 per cent of advanced ovarian cancer. It may be raised with other tumours such as pancreas, lung, breast and colorectal. Benign conditions may also have raised levels: menstruation, pelvic inflammatory disease, endometriosis, pregnancy, tuberculosis, pericarditis and liver cirrhosis.

208.

A. **False.**   MSAFP levels are low, and levels of unconjugated oestriol and human chorionic gonadotrophin (hCG) are raised.

B. **False.**   Levels of unconjugated oestriol and hCG are also low in trisomy 18.

C. **True.**

D. **True.**   An elevated MSAFP denotes a high-risk pregnancy and is a marker for later pre-eclampsia or intra-uterine growth retardation.

E. **True.**

F. **True.**

G. **True.**

H. **True.**

Causes of raised AFP

First-trimester bleeding; intra-uterine death; twins; abdominal wall defects; congenital nephrosis; Turner's syndrome; epidermolysis bullosa; rhesus disease and renal agenesis and later pre-eclampsia and intra-uterine growth retardation.

209.

A. **True.** Primary dysmenorrhoea occurs in the absence of an organic or psychological cause for painful periods. On the other hand, secondary dysmenorrhoea always has an underlying cause.

B. **False.** The pain usually starts some hours before the menstrual flow and disappears within 2–3 days.

C. **False.** Prostaglandin is associated with uterine cramping as well as hypersensitization of the pain terminus.

D. **False.** On the contrary, this method is well proven and helps 90 per cent of these patients.

E. **True.** This is thought to be the case. Other exacerbating factors include a lack of sleep, and stress.

F. **False.** The condition usually occurs in the teenage years, whereas secondary dysmenorrhoea usually starts during adult life.

210.

A. **False.** There is a greater risk of pulmonary oedema and other side effects in multiple (twin) pregnancy.

B. **False.** Blood sugar and blood pressure must be monitored carefully when tocolytics are in use. Pyrexia is not a recognized side effect of beta-mimetic therapy.

C. **True.** Injudicious use of beta-sympathomimetic drugs and corticosteroids can precipitate acute pulmonary oedema – strict control of fluid balance is necessary.

211.

A. **True.**

B. **True.** Echogenic bowel occurs in less than 1 per cent of pregnancies. The bowel looks bright, being similar in echogenicity to the spine/ribs. It can be seen in up to 13 per cent of fetuses with cystic fibrosis.

C. **True.** Echogenic bowel is detected in 3 per cent of fetuses with aneuploidy.

D. **True.** In about 85 per cent of cases, there is no associated pathology.

212.

A. **True.** That is, more than 42 weeks.

B. **True.** And overgrown nails, abundant scalp hair, scaphoid abdomen and minimal subcutaneous fat.

C. **True.** However, at 37–42 weeks' gestation antepartum deaths constitute two-thirds of perinatal mortality.

213.

A. **False.**

B. **False.**

C. **True.**

D. **False.**

E. **True.**

Placenta praevia

The incidence of placenta praevia is 1 in 200, and the mortality rate in the developed world is 0.03 per cent. Vaginal ultrasound is the best method of diagnosis and has been shown to be safer and more sensitive than abdominal ultrasound. If the placental edge is 2 cm or closer to the internal os, the baby is best delivered by Caesarean section. The risk of placenta accreta is increased 2000-fold in the presence of praevia, and increased again if there is a lower uterine segment scar.

Ref: Placenta praevia: diagnosis and management Guideline 27. RCOG 2001.

214.

A. **False.** The correct figure is 60 ± 20 mL.

B. **False.** Only 10 per cent of patients are anovulatory.

C. **False.** The opposite is **True.** Polyps, fibroids and adenomyosis are associated with a lower rate of success.

D. **True.**

E. **False.** The diagnosis is made only after hysterectomy.

215.

A. **False.** The term describes abnormal bleeding in the absence of organic pathology or systemic disease.

B. **True.** Only 10 per cent of DUB is thought to be ovulatory.

C. **False.** This investigation is generally reserved for patients in whom medical treatment has failed or where other lesions are suspected, e.g. endometrial polyp.

D. **True.** Anovulatory menorrhagia is easier to treat and usually responds to progestogen therapy.

E. **False.** Progestogen therapy is not recommended in this situation. There is little benefit, and side effects include breast tenderness and water retention.

F. **False.** Additional contraception is warranted and advised.

216.

A. **True.**

B. **True.**

C. **True.**

D. **False.**

Human papillomavirus (HPV)

DNA probing has identified more than 70 types of HPV, and types 6, 11, 16, 18, 31, 33 and 35 seem to be closely associated with anogenital infection. Increasing awareness of how certain types are linked to anogenital cancer means that HPV is a potential threat to health, rather than being just a nuisance STD.

A new treatment for external genital and perianal warts, Aldara® cream, has recently been approved by the FDA. Aldara (imiquimod) cream is the newest in a class of drugs known as 'immune response modifiers', and represents the first new therapeutic approach to genital warts in 5 years.

Aldara is a vanishing cream applied by the patient, in the privacy of the home, and is available on prescription only.

217.

A. **False.** Multiple sexual partners and early intercourse are among the many risk factors for cervical disease.

218.

A. **True.** It drains into the posterior aspect of the introitus. Normally, the glands are small and not palpable.
B. **True.** Infection causes the cyst contents to become purulent.
C. **False.** Small, asymptomatic cysts do not require any treatment unless recurrent or infected.
D. **True.** Organisms implicated include *E. coli*, *Proteus* and *Neisseria gonorrhoea*.
E. **False.** Trauma and congenital stenosis may cause cyst and/or abscess formation.

219.

A. **True.**
B. **False.** Lymphogranuloma venereum is caused by *Chlamydia trachomatis* serovars L1, L2 and L3.
C. **True.** With gross distortion of the perineal tissues.

220.

A. **False.**
B. **False.** There is no evidence to support this at the present time. Nd:Yag lasers and KtP-532 lasers are used. It is suggested that more precise tissue destruction allows healing without adhesions, and also minimizes damage to surrounding tissues.
C. **False.**
D. **True.**
E. **True.**

Progestogens used in the treatment of endometriosis

Progestogens alone:

- Oral medroxprogesterone acetate.
- Injectable medroxprogesterone acetate.
- Megestrol acetate.
- Dydrogesterone.

Progestogens in combination with oestrogens:

- Desogestrel.
- Cyproterone acetate.

221.

A. **True.** The progesterone-only pill (POP) is a good choice in situations where oestrogen is contraindicated, such as patients with serious medical conditions (diabetes with vascular disease, severe systemic lupus erythematosus (SLE) and cardiovascular disease).

B. **True.**

Contraception for diabetic women:

- All women of childbearing age need contraceptive advice if pregnancy is not intended.
- Barrier methods/low-dose oral contraceptive if low arterial risk.
- Stop contraception only when adequate control is achieved.
- Sterilization may be preferable when the family is complete.
- Emergency contraception can be used by diabetic women.

222.

A. **True.** Translocation 14:21 accounts for 2 per cent, other translocations for 2 per cent, and mosaicism 1 per cent.

B. **True.** Individual incidences of Down's syndrome (trisomy 21) depend on maternal age.

C. **False.** The mean IQ is approximately 50 in Down's syndrome children, and corresponds to severe mental retardation.

D. **True.** Congenital heart disease lesions associated with Down's syndrome include atrioventricular canal defects, ventricular septal defects, patent ductus arteriosus, primum atrioseptal defect and tetralogy of Fallot.

E. **False.** Gastro-intestinal atresias are common, especially duodenal atresia, and there is early dementia with similarities to Alzheimer's disease.

F. **False.** 20 per cent of babies die before the age of 1 year, but 45 per cent reach 60 years of age.

Down's syndrome

The diagnosis can generally be made shortly after birth. The ten principal features are:

• Hypotonia	80 per cent
• Poor Moro reflex	85 per cent
• Hyperflexibility of joints	80 per cent
• Excess skin on back of neck	80 per cent
• Flat face	90 per cent
• Slanted palpebral fissures	80 per cent
• Anomalous auricles	60 per cent
• Dysplasia of pelvis	70 per cent
• Dysplasia of middle phalanx, 5th finger	60 per cent
• Simian crease	45 per cent

The incidence of Down's syndrome increases with advancing maternal age, although the overall incidence is 1:660 newborns.

- 20 years – 1:2000
- 30 years – 1:900
- 35 years – 1:350
- 36 years – 1:240
- 38 years – 1:180
- 40 years – 1:100
- 44 years – 1:40

223.
A. **True.** In early pregnancy choroid plexus cysts (up to 10 mm in diameter) can be a normal finding. They are often bilateral, thought to be developmental in origin, and usually disappear by 24 weeks' gestation.
B. **False.** Choroid plexus cysts are associated with trisomy 18 (Edward's syndrome) and trisomy 13 (Patu's syndrome), but not associated with trisomy 21 (Down's syndrome).

224.
A. **True.**
B. **False.** It indicates stage II.
C. **False.** The correct figure is 70–75 per cent.

Clinical staging of carcinoma of cervix:

- Stage 0 = Intraepithelial carcinoma.
- Stage I = Invasive carcinoma confined to the cervix.
- Stage Ia1: No lesion visible at clinical examination, and stromal invasion is less than 3 mm (microinvasion).
- Stage Ia2: Stromal invasion between 3–5 mm with maximum lateral spread of 7 mm.
- Stage Ib: All other stage I lesions.
- Stage Ib1: Clinical lesions no greater than 4 cm in size.
- Stage Ib2: Clinical lesions greater than 4 cm in size.
- Stage II = The carcinoma extends beyond the cervix but not to the pelvic side wall, and/or the upper two-thirds of the vagina are involved.
- Stage IIa: No parametrial involvement.
- Stage IIb: Obvious parametrial involvement.
- Stage III = The carcinoma extends to the pelvic side wall, and/or the lower one-third of the vagina is involved. Presence of hydronephrosis or non-functioning kidney.
- Stage IIIa: No extension to the pelvic wall, but involvement of the lower third of vagina.
- Stage IIIb: Extension to the pelvic wall or hydronephrosis or non-functioning kidney.
- Stage IV = The carcinoma extends beyond the true pelvis, or involves the bladder or rectum (bullous oedema is excluded).
- Stage IVa: Spread of tumour onto adjacent pelvic organ.
- Stage IVb: Spread to distant organs.

225.
A. **True.** In addition, steroids should be given, as the greatest risk is of prematurity.
B. **True.** And delays delivery. No effect has yet been shown demonstrating an improvement in perinatal mortality. Patients identified as carriers of Group B haemolytic *Streptococcus* (GBS) should receive intrapartum antibiotics.
C. **False.** Decreases the risk by about 50 per cent. Development of respiratory distress syndrome and incidence of fetal/neonatal death are not affected.

The ORACLE trial

The role of antibiotics has been clarified by the ORACLE trial (Overview of the Role of Antibiotics in Curtailing Labour and Early Delivery). After preterm, premature rupture of the membranes, antibiotics given to the mother reduce maternal infection, fetal infection, the number of babies born after 48 h and after 7 days, and the number of babies requiring surfactant. Macrolide antibiotics are recommended (e.g. erythromycin) as beta-lactam antibiotics (e.g. augmentin) increase the likelihood of neonatal necrotizing enterocolitis. (*Cochrane Database* 2001; **4**: CD001058)

226.
A. **False.** Infertility is an issue for 30–40 per cent of women with endometriosis. This may be due, in part at least, to anatomical distortion secondary to the disease.
B. **False.**
C. **True.**
D. **False.**

Mechanisms of infertility in patients with mild-to-moderate endometriosis:

- Changes in peritoneal fluid.
  - Increase in volume, presence of interleukins and tumour necrosis factor, increased prostaglandin levels and increased number of macrophages.
- Ovulation disorders.
  - Anovulation, hyperprolactinaemia, abnormal follicular rupture, luteal phase defect, luteinized unruptured follicles.
- Pelvic pain.
- Immunological abnormalities.
  - T cells, antigen-specific B-cell activation, anti-endometrial antibodies, non-specific B-cell activation.
- Spontaneous abortion.
- Implantation.

227.
A. **True.** Little is known of the aetiology of vulval cancer. Cigarette smoking is associated, and the patient may have had cervical intraepithelial or invasive disease. A viral factor has been suggested by the detection of antigens induced by herpes simplex virus (HSV) 2 and of DNA from type 16/18 HPV (human papillomavirus) in VIN (vulval intraepithelial neoplasm), and also by the association of a history of genital warts with vulval cancer.
B. **True.** The condition itself is considered benign, but it may progress to malignancy in approximately 3 per cent of cases.

228.

A. **True.** And post-coital aching.

B. **False.** The pain is variable in nature and location, radiates through to the back or down the legs, and is exacerbated on standing and relieved on lying down.

C. **True.** A randomized controlled trial of medroxyprogesterone acetate 30–50 mg/day showed positive results. Other treatment modalities include ultrasound, psychological intervention, laparoscopy and total abdominal hysterectomy (TAH) and bilateral salpingo-oophorectomy (BSO). The following are not considered useful: TAH with ovarian conservation, presacral neurectomy and laparoscopic uterosacral nerve ablation (LUNA).

229.

A. **False.** COCP may be used as post-coital contraception.

B. **False.** Mifepristone produces changes in the histology of the endometrium. There are three major characteristics of its action which are important: a long half-life; high affinity for the progesterone receptor; and active metabolites.

C. **False.** It is two doses of 0.75 mg 12 h apart. It is a suitable method for those women who cannot take oestrogen.

D. **False.** The combined method is not suitable for women with a history of thrombosis, active acute porphyria, and for those with focal migraine at the time of presentation.

Post-coital contraception

Hormonal methods for emergency contraception use either levonorgestrel alone or combined with ethinylestradiol. They are both effective if taken within 72 h of unprotected intercourse, although taking the first dose within 12 h significantly increases its efficacy. Levonelle-2 containing 750 micrograms of levonorgestrel has replaced the combined hormonal (Yuzpe) method containing ethinylestradiol 50 micrograms and levonorgestrel 250 micrograms as the first choice for emergency contraception.

230.

A. **False.** HPV is found in a high proportion of squamous cell carcinomas of the vulva, but no causative mechanism has been proven.

B. **False.** Over 80 per cent are squamous cell carcinomas. Vulval adenocarcinomas have an origin in the Bartholin's gland.

C. **True.** This is one of the nodes within the femoral canal, which may be affected in vulval carcinoma.

D. **True.** Surgical treatment is preferred as radio- and chemotherapy are of unproven benefit.

E. **False.** Chemotherapy is only of value when used in conjunction with radiotherapy. The role of this combination is under trial with respect to advanced squamous carcinoma.

> ### Clinical staging of carcinoma of vulva:
>
> - Stage I: Lesions 2 cm or less confined to the vulva or perineum. No lymph node metastases.
> - Stage Ia: As above with stromal invasion no greater than 1 mm.
> - Stage Ib: Stromal invasion more than 1 mm.
> - Stage II: Lesions confined to the vulva and/or perineum with a diameter >2 cm and no lymph node metastases.
> - Stage III: Lesions of any size extending to the lower urethra, vagina or anus and/or unilateral node metastases.
> - Stage IVa: Lesions invading upper urethra, bladder, rectum or pelvic bone with or without bilateral positive groin nodes, regardless of extent of primary.
> - Stage IVb: Any distant metastases including pelvic lymph nodes.

231.

A. **True.** Hysterectomy is the most frequently performed major gynaecological operation on women of reproductive age.

B. **True.** Less than 80 mL per month.

C. **False.** In the majority of cases there is no organic disease, and the bleeding is described as dysfunctional. Dysfunctional uterine bleeding is associated with anovulation in 10–20 per cent of women.

D. **False.** 20 per cent.

232.

A. **True.** Reductions in blood loss of up to 50 per cent have been reported using tranexamic acid. Mefenamic acid inhibits prostaglandins.

B. **True.**

C. **True.** While caution has been advised in the administration of fibrinolytic inhibitors for menorrhagia, no increase in the incidence of thromboembolic disease was seen in a recent Scandinavian trial.

D. **True.** Mefenamic acid and tranexamic acid reduce menstrual blood loss by about 25 per cent and 50 per cent, respectively.

E. **True.**

233.

A. **False.** Bromocriptine is effective in more than 90 per cent of patients. Indications for treating microprolactinomas (having a diameter <10 mm on computed tomography brain scanning) include menstrual disturbance, infertility, oestrogen deficiency, troublesome galactorrhoea, decreased libido and dizziness.

B. **False.** Bromocriptine intolerance can be reduced by starting with a small night-time dose taken with food before retiring.

C. **False.** 1.25 mg.

D. **True.** Carbergoline is a dopamine agonist, reportedly with fewer side effects than bromocriptine.

Bromocriptine and carbergoline

Bromocriptine is a stimulant of dopamine receptors in the brain, and inhibits release of prolactin by the pituitary gland. It is used in the treatment of galactorrhoea, cyclical benign breast disease, prolactinomas and, as it inhibits the release of growth hormone, it is sometimes used in the treatment of acromegaly.

Doses:

- Suppression of lactation: 2.5 mg on day 1 (prevention) or daily for 2–3 days for suppression, then 2.5 mg twice daily for 14 days.
- Prolactinoma: initially 1.0–1.25 mg at bedtime, increasing gradually to 5 mg every 6 h.

Carbergoline has similar action and uses as bromocriptine.

Doses:
- Prevention of lactation: 1 mg on day 1 as a single dose.
- Suppression of established lactation: 250 micrograms every 12 h for 2 days.
- Hyperprolactinaemic disorders: 500 micrograms weekly; increase at monthly intervals in steps of 500 micrograms until optimal therapeutic response.

234.
A. **True.**   Sickle-cell disease can be diagnosed antenatally by chorionic villus sampling (CVS) or amniocentesis. Crises may be precipitated by infection, dehydration, hypoxia, cold and venous stasis.
B. **True.**   There is also an increased risk of fetal loss, intra-uterine growth retardation and prematurity.
C. **False.**   It is coded on chromosome 16 by two genes. The beta-thalassaemia genes are carried on chromosome 16. Haemoglobin S, for sickle-cell disease, is also carried on chromosome 16.
D. **False.**   More than 150.

235.
A. **False.**
B. **False.**
C. **False.**
D. **False.**

Complications of cervical cancer:

- Pyometra due to obstruction of the cervical canal and infection; therefore it is common.
- Vesicovaginal and vesicocervical fistulas.
- Rectovaginal fistulas (rare in untreated cases).
- Hydronephrosis and pyonephrosis caused by ureteric obstruction.
- Uraemia; this is caused by renal failure due to combination of infection and ureteric obstruction.

236.

A. **True.** A large tongue and kidneys, microcephaly and small exomphalos are characteristic.

B. **False.** Azoospermia is the rule in cystic fibrosis.

C. **False.** Antenatal screening for cystic fibrosis is possible, with chorionic villus sampling (CVS) being performed if both parents are gene carriers. 1 in 20 of the population is a carrier, resulting in a disease incidence of 1 in 2000 live-born infants.

D. **False.** The development of a cystic hygroma is multifactorial; it probably develops from a defect in the formation of lymphatic vessels. This results from a failure of the venous system and lymphatic system to connect; thus lymph fluid accumulates in the jugular lymph sacs.

237.

A. **False.** They are effective in 75 per cent of women.

B. **False.** Reductions in blood loss of up to 50 per cent have been reported using TA in women with dysfunctional uterine bleeding (DUB), or in those with bleeding associated with fibroids or coagulation defects.

C. **False.** Inhibition of uterine prostaglandin production reduces menstrual blood loss by 20–50 per cent in about three-quarters of women with menorrhagia. The beneficial effect of mefenamic acid specifically appears to persist.

D. **True.** Fibrinolytic inhibitors appear to be more effective, but adverse effects are more common.

238.

A. **False.** Various methods involving the use of rollerball, radiofrequency ablation and transcervical resection are now well-accepted methods of treatment of menorrhagia.

B. **False.** Endometrial ablation offers a less invasive surgical approach, but its irreversibility means women wishing to retain reproductive function are not suitable for the procedure.

C. **True.** Over 80 per cent of women will become amenorrhoeic or hypomenorrhoeic following hysteroscopic surgery. However, up to 20 per cent eventually request further treatment.

D. **True.** Hysteroscopic operations are comparable with hysterectomy in terms of freedom from major complications. However, a much-reduced incidence of minor morbidity, mostly infection, and a much shorter postoperative recovery period was demonstrated in the hysteroscopic group.

E. **True.** Although some isolated reports are to the contrary, randomized controlled trials show cyclical pain to be decreased after such treatments.

F. **True.**

G. **False.** The figure is 20 per cent.

H. **True.** Combined HRT is essential as some endometrium persists, even in amenorrhoeic women.

239.

A. **True.**

B. **True.** The average time required for progression from hyperplasia to carcinoma is approximately 5 years.

C. **False.** 1–3 per cent.

D. **False.** If atypia is present, 20–25 per cent of cases will progress to carcinoma within 1 year.

E. **True.**

F. **False.** Provera 5 mg/day for 10 days/month for 1 year is advised.

> **Risk factors for endometrial hyperplasia and endometrial cancer:**
> - Menstrual cycle irregularity.
> - Obesity.
> - Infertility.
> - Nulliparity.
> - Age >40 years.
> - Family history of colon cancer.

240.

A. **False.** About 25 per cent of total testosterone derives from the ovaries, a further 25 per cent from the adrenals (driven by adrenocorticotrophic hormone – ACTH), and the remaining 50 per cent from peripheral conversion of androstenedione in skin, fat and liver.

B. **True.** Only free testosterone is thought to be biologically active. Within the skin, the enzyme 5a-reductase transforms testosterone into dihydrotestosterone, a very potent androgen.

C. **False.** Commonly ovarian, much less commonly, adrenal.

D. **True.** There are two main hypotheses for the development of PCOD: (1) Adrenal hyperandrogenaemia; (2) Hyperinsulinaemia secondary to insulin receptor dysfunction.

241.

A. **True.** Replacement involves glucocorticoid therapy, and mineralocorticoid is also often required.

B. **True.** And plasma renin activity.

C. **True.** Inheritance is in an autosomal recessive manner.

Congenital adrenal hyperplasia (CAH)

The commonest enzyme defect is 21-hydroxylase deficiency which interferes with the conversion of 17-alpha-hydroxyprogesterone to desoxycortisol and with the conversion of progesterone to desoxycorticosterone. The resulting cortisol deficiency leads to increased adrenocorticotrophine hormone (ACTH) production, overstimulation of the adrenal, large amounts of androgens and masculinization of the fetus.

242.

A. **True.** Physiological hyperprolactinaemia can be caused by sleep, pregnancy, lactation, stress, and renal or hepatic dysfunction.

B. **True.**

Prolactin

High levels in the fetus decline rapidly after birth. Levels are higher in girls than boys after puberty, and are slightly higher in the luteal phase of the cycle.

Levels are increased steadily during pregnancy, reaching values 10–20 times those in the non-pregnant state. In the absence of suckling, levels return to normal 2–3 weeks after delivery.

243.

A. True.

B. True.

C. **False.** Bromocriptine is safe in pregnancy and not associated with an increased risk of miscarriage, congenital anomalies or multiple pregnancy.

D. False.

E. False.

244.

A. **False.** The management of the preterm breech fetus in labour remains a problem. Caesarean section is used increasingly in an effort to improve the condition of the neonate at birth. It is not clear from examination of the scientific evidence and consideration of the balance between fetal or neonatal and maternal risk that this is the optimum mode of delivery. Even at Caesarean section, a baby with very low birth weight is susceptible to trauma. This difficulty can be avoided by a classical incision into the uterus. However, this will increase maternal morbidity from sepsis, blood loss and risk of rupture in a subsequent pregnancy. The high neonatal mortality rate at less than 28 weeks and the high maternal morbidity of classical Caesarean section may mean that vaginal delivery should be chosen for the very preterm baby.

B. **True.** The following are more common during a vaginal breech delivery: cerebellar damage and ataxic cerebral palsy; intraventricular and periventricular damage secondary to haemorrhage or ischaemia; widespread limb and body bruising secondary to a traumatic delivery; damage to internal organs; entrapment of the aftercoming head with consequent hypoxia; and mechanical stress and prolapse of the cord (commonest in a footling breech). All of the above problems may also be encountered during abdominal delivery.

C. **True.** An ultrasound scan confirms presentation and excludes fetal abnormality. In addition, fetal weight is estimated and placental site determined.

D. **True.** A senior obstetrician should attend vaginal delivery if possible. The anaesthetist and paediatrician should also be in attendance. If the head becomes entrapped behind an incompletely dilated cervix, it should first be carefully flexed. Failing this, the cervix should be incised at 4 and 8 o'clock, after which the head should deliver with ease.

E. **False.** Most of the published data about the optimum mode of delivery of the preterm breech baby are observational and retrospective, leading to serious bias that tends to favour Caesarean section rather than vaginal delivery. The preterm breech baby delivered vaginally tends to be lighter, of a lower gestational age, and in a poorer condition. Even with more statistically sophisticated techniques to control these confounding variables, no clear consensus emerges from the data. Two other randomized trials of the mode of delivery of the preterm breech baby produced no reliable conclusions because data were analysed by actual mode of delivery rather than the policy allocated. (See RCOG guidelines.)

245.

A. **True.** CHD affects about 5–8:1000 live births.

B. **True.** CHD is associated with a 15 per cent increase in the risk of aneuploidy.

C. **False.** Down's syndrome (trisomy 21) and Edward's syndrome (trisomy 18) are the most common aneuploidies associated with CHD.

D. **True.** Other factors which have greater risk for CHD are:
non-immune hydrops fetalis; extracardiac anomalies (20 per cent); either parent with CHD (mother) or sibling with CHD (2–6 per cent); diabetes mellitus (3 per cent, or less, if well controlled in the first trimester); fetal arrhythmia; and drugs such as lithium and anticonvulsants.

E. **False.** It will only identify 25–40 per cent of all major cardiac abnormalities. Viewing the aorta and pulmonary artery increases the sensitivity to greater than 60 per cent.

246.

A. **False.** Kallman's syndrome is a condition where there is inadequate release of GnRH and subsequent amenorrhoea. It is characterized by anosmia. Sexual development is grossly retarded.

B. **False.**

C. **True.**

D. **True.**

E. **False.**

247.

A. **True.** Bisphosphanates have a high affinity for bone, and their major effect is to inhibit osteoclast function and recruitment. As a result, the imbalance in turnover is normalized and this eventually leads to an increase in bone mass.

B. **True.**

C. **True.**

D. **False.** A combination of 800 IU of vitamin D and 1200 mg calcium in elderly postmenopausal women increased bone mineral density and resulted in a significant reduction in hip (23 per cent) and non-vertebral fractures (17 per cent).

E. **True.** Raloxifene is a SERM (selective estrogen receptor modulator). It has the desirable effects of oestrogen, such as increasing bone density and creating a beneficial lipid profile without the detrimental effects on breast and endometrium.

Products licensed for the prevention and treatment of osteoporosis

Bisphosphonates:

- Etidronate: 400 mg daily for 14 days, followed by Calcit (calcium carbonate) 1.25 g for 76 days.
- Risedronate: 5 mg daily.
- Alendronate: 5 mg daily for prevention; 10 mg daily or 70 mg weekly for treatment of osteoporosis.
- Alendronate: 70 mg weekly.

SERMS:

- Raloxifene: 60 mg daily.

Calcitonin:

- Salcatonin: 100 units daily intramuscularly or subcutaneously for 28 days.

248.
A. True.
B. True.
C. False.
D. False.
E. False.

249.
A. True.
B. False. Twice as common.
C. True. Maternal genes are not expressed.
D. False. Two paternal and one maternal.
E. False. Dramatically increased, 1:3 pregnancies.

250.
A. True. And a decreased risk of necrotizing enterocolitis.
B. False. The regulation of surfactant production and its release is still not clear. Also, the mechanism of cortisol effect is still not clear.
C. False. TRH in combination with corticosteroids improves the efficacy of antenatal corticosteroids, but the side effects of TRH restrict its use.
D. True.
E. False. Between 24 h and 7 days.
F. False.
G. False.

251.
A. **True.**
B. **False.** There is a theoretical risk of pyometra. Oral oestrogen 5 days prior to the attempted removal may facilitate the procedure.

252.
A. **True.** The intra-uterine gestation sac is first seen at 29 days (menstrual age) when it appears as a 2–3 mm echo-free structure surrounded by the hyperechoic trophoblastic ring. It is almost always located eccentrically within the uterine cavity.
B. **False.** In multiple pregnancies, the serum hCG level will be significantly higher than 1000 IU/L before the gestation sacs are seen.
C. **True.** In the remainder, there are three sonographic features of tubal pregnancy. First, the demonstration of a live embryo within a gestational sac in the adnexae – 'the bagel sign'. The second transvaginal ultrasound picture of tubal pregnancy is that of a poorly defined tubal ring, possibly containing echogenic structures. Typically, the pouch of Douglas also contains fluid and/or blood. These features are consistent with a tubal pregnancy that is aborting. The third typical sonographic picture is the presence of varying amounts of fluid in the pouch of Douglas representing bleeding from the tubal pregnancy.

253.
A. **True.** The vault of the skull and cerebral cortex are absent. Spina bifida includes:
Anencephaly: the vault of the skull and cerebral cortex are absent.
Meningocele: dura and arachnoid mater bulge through a defect in the spine.
Myelomeningocele: the central canal of the cord is exposed.
Encephalocele: there is a bony defect in the cranial vault through which a dura mater sac (+ brain tissue) protrudes.
B. **False.** Neural tube defects (NTDs) are more common in Scotland and Ireland (3:1000), but have a lower incidence in England (2:1000). In USA, Japan, Canada and Africa the incidence is much less (<1:1000).
C. **True.** The incidence is 1:10 if two or more siblings are affected, and 1:25 if one parent is affected.
D. **True.** Hydrocephalus occurs in about 90 per cent of fetuses with spina bifida. Spina bifida alone has a better prognosis.
E. **True.** Blunting of the sinciput (the lemon sign) and a banana-shaped cerebellum (Arnold–Chiari malformation) or absent cerebellum are markers for spina bifida.
F. **False.** Folic acid, 5 mg/day orally, from before conception reduces the risk of recurrence. A preconceptual prophylactic dose of 400 micrograms/day is recommended for all other pregnant women.

254.
A. **True.** The COCP protects against ovarian cancer and should be recommended to women with a family history of ovarian cancer.
B. **False.**
C. **False.** The risk of developing ovarian cancer is decreased by approximately 40 per cent.
D. **True.** A decrease of 50 per cent is seen after 3 years of COCP use.

Protective benefits of COCP

The COCP protects against endometriosis. It also provides protection against pelvic inflammatory disease. Its relationship with breast cancer and cervical intraepithelial neoplasia is more controversial. There is some epidemiological evidence that it will increase the risk of breast cancer.

255.
A. **True.** The incidence increases with age. The COCP is protective.
B. **True.** The risk of ovarian cancer is doubled in patients suffering from breast cancer.
C. **False.** Stage I disease is confined to the ovaries; stage II involves spread beyond the ovaries.
D. **False.** The 5-year survival rate of patients with stage I disease is 80 per cent, while the correct figure for stage IV disease is only 25 per cent.
E. **False.** These tumours are epithelial tumours with histological features of cancer but excellent prognosis.

Staging of ovarian cancer:

- Stage I: Growth limited to the ovaries.
- Stage Ia: Only one ovary involved, no ascites (subgroups: capsule not ruptured; capsule ruptured).
- Stage Ib: Both ovaries involved, no ascites (subgroups: as above).
- Stage Ic: One or both ovaries involved plus ascites or with malignant cells in peritoneal washing (subgroups: as above).
- Stage IIa: Extension/metastases to uterus/tubes.
- Stage IIb: Extension to other pelvic tissue.
- Stage IIc: As IIa/b with ascites or positive peritoneal washing.
- Stage III: Growth involving one or both ovaries with intraperitoneal metastasis.
- Stage IV: Growth involving one or both ovaries with distant metastasis.

256.
A. **False.** The definition is accurate except for the gestation described. The correct figure is 37 weeks' gestation.
B. **False.** The majority of cases are idiopathic. However, urinary tract infection, dehydration and systemic infection may contribute.
C. **True.** This is one of many risk factors including chorioamnionitis, smoking, infections, polyhydramnios and advanced maternal age.
D. **False.** 5–10 per cent of pregnancies.
E. **False.** The major problem is pulmonary immaturity and intraventricular haemorrhage. These infants are at greater risk of sepsis and necrotizing enterocolitis.
F. **False.** Tocolytics should be used up to 34 weeks' gestation. They are justified for at least 48 h to allow intra-uterine transfer and steroid administration.

257.
A. **True.** Peritoneal healing differs from that of other epithelial tissues. Mesothelial cells migrate into a supportive matrix and simultaneously initiate multiple sites of repair.
B. **True.**
C. **False.**
D. **True.** Suturing can lead to ischaemia, which suppresses normal fibrinolytic activity. Unabsorbed fibrin becomes stabilized, infiltrated by fibroblasts and ultimately organized into permanent adhesions.
E. **False.**

258.
A. **True.** This produces vaporization of the tissue with minimal coagulation.
B. **False.** The pulse pressure is decreased by this mechanism.
C. **False.** Such stretching is associated with a bradycardia.
D. **True.** Traumatic injury is more likely to cause haemorrhage, whereas thermal injury is associated with full-thickness bowel injury and necrosis.
E. **True.** This corresponds with the level of L4. Caution is advised where the Trendelenberg position is effected.

259.
A. **True.** In an embryo that has developed up to 5 mm, loss of viability occurs in 7.2 per cent. Loss rates drop to 3.3 per cent for embryos of 6–10 mm.
B. **True.** The reliability of ultrasonography in the detection of complete miscarriage is high: 98 per cent of patients with an empty uterus who do not need any further intervention are correctly identified.
C. **True.** About one-third of normal embryos with a crown–rump length <5 mm have no demonstrable cardiac activity. Thus, the diagnosis of missed miscarriage should not be made in embryos smaller than this.
D. **True.** Or the crown–rump length greater than 6 mm.
E. **True.** Recent findings suggest that the most likely explanation is the early demise and resorption of the embryo with persistence of placental tissue rather than a pregnancy originally without an embryo.

Early pregnancy

The gestational sac diameter increases in size from 2–4 mm by 5.0 weeks, and is 5 mm by 5.2 weeks. A gestational sac of 2, 5, 10, 20 and 25 mm diameter roughly corresponds to a pregnancy of about 4, 5, 6, 7 and 8 weeks from the last monthly period (LMP), respectively.

The gestational sac volume increases from 1 mL at 6 weeks to 31 mL at 10 weeks and 100 mL at 13 weeks.

In normal pregnancy, the sac diameter increases by 1.2 mm/day.

260.

A. **True.** Prophylaxis should be reserved for those patients with additional risk factors, e.g. thrombophilias, recurrent thrombosis and post-thrombotic venous insufficiency.

B. **False.** Start 4–6 weeks before the gestational time when the previous event occurred.

C. **True.** Paradoxically, yes! Thrombocytopenia secondary to prolonged antenatal low-dose heparin has been associated with thrombosis, which is difficult to treat.

D. **False.** 4.6 per cent. Heparin, however, does not cross the placenta. Central nervous system abnormalities secondary to warfarin treatment occur even where control is good. It is thought that the lesions occur after damage to larger blood vessels that results in infarction of the developing brain.

E. **False.** There is a risk of anaphylactoid reaction to Dextran 70.

F. **True.**

G. **True.** Because of the risk of spinal haematoma.

H. **False.** The guidelines say 4–6 h.

I. **True.** But there are no significant changes in postoperative haemoglobin levels or blood transfusion requirements.

261.

A. **True.**

B. **True.**

C. **False.** 10 years.

D. **False.** The incidence is 15–20 per cent. In Africa, where breast-feeding is the norm, the rate is about 25–35 per cent.

E. **True.** Both emergency and elective.

RNA-containing viruses:

- Picornaviruses: enteroviruses (coxsackie, ECHO, polio) and rhinoviruses (common cold).
- Reoviruses (including rotaviruses): respiratory tract infections and diarrhoea in children.
- Myxoviruses: influenza.
- Paramyxoviruses: mumps, para-influenza, measles, respiratory syncytial virus.
- Arboviruses (arthropod borne): encephalitis, yellow fever, dengue, sandfly fever.
- Rhabdoviruses: rabies.
- Retroviruses: HIV, HTLV 1.

262.

A. **True.**

B. **False.** Not recommended until 6 h have elapsed since the last dose of prostaglandin.

C. **False.** The maximum licensed rate is 0.02 milliunits per minute, but the maximum recommended rate is 0.032 milliunits per minute.

263.

A. **True.** The success rate is about 20 per cent. However, there is a higher risk of spontaneous abortion, multiple pregnancy (25 per cent), pregnancy-induced hypertension, preterm labour, breech presentation, small-for-dates baby and antepartum haemorrhage. There is no increase in the incidence of congenital abnormalities.

B. **False.** The embryo is returned to the endometrial cavity as might be expected.

C. **True.** Thus the risks and expenses of IVF are decreased.

D. **True.** Oocyte retrieval is completed via transabdominal, transvaginal and transcervical routes, and ultrasound guidance is used in most centres. Every effort is made to avoid the bowel, but occasionally it will be punctured.

264.

A. **True.** Anticholinergic drugs produce competitive blockade of acetylcholine receptors at postganglionic parasympathetic receptors.

B. **False.** Anticholinergic drugs are not specific to the bladder, and produce antimuscarinic effects in many other organs.

C. **False.** Blurring of vision may be caused by transient paralysis of the iris and of the ciliary muscle of the lens controlling accommodation. Eye pain may indicate glaucoma, and the drug should be stopped.

D. **False.** Often, the manufacturer's stated dose is too high, and it is worth titrating the dose upwards until symptoms are controlled.

E. **True.**

Anticholinergic drugs

Anticholinergic drugs (antimuscarinic) are used to treat urinary frequency; they relax the detrusor muscle and increase bladder capacity by diminishing unstable detrusor contractions.

Oxybutynin directly relaxes urinary smooth muscle, but has a high level of side effects, which limits its use.

Contraindications: myasthenia gravia, glaucoma, significant bladder outflow obstruction or urinary retention, severe ulcerative colitis, toxic megacolon, and gastro-intestinal obstruction or intestinal atony.

Side effects: dry mouth, constipation, blurred vision, drowsiness, nausea, vomiting, abdominal discomfort, difficulty in micturition, palpitations, skin reactions, headache, diarrhoea, angioedema, arrhythmias and tachycardia.

Also central nervous system stimulation, such as restlessness, disorientation, hallucination and convulsions.

265.

A. **False.** It is the second commonest cause in women and accounts for 30–40 per cent. The definition is otherwise **True.**
B. **True.** GSI accounts for approximately 50 per cent of cases referred for urodynamics.
C. **True.**
D. **False.** A decreased maximum flow rate may indicate outflow obstruction or inadequate detrusor function.
E. **False.** GSI can only be diagnosed indirectly at urodynamics, and it is important to have a well-trained operator who can interpret the trace and label it correctly.

266.

A. **True.** This is thought to be due to the increasing incidence of salpingitis, treated successfully with antibiotics but leaving residual tubal damage.
B. **True.** Other risk factors include previous infection and tubal surgery.
C. **False.** While the majority of ectopic pregnancies occur in the Fallopian tube, the ampulla is the commonest site.
D. **False.** Elevated temperature is not a usual sign of ectopic pregnancy. More common are abdominal pain and vaginal staining.
E. **False.** It is a useful agent due to its action on DNA synthesis.

Ectopic pregnancy

Ectopic pregnancy is often difficult to diagnose, but can have catastrophic results if missed. It should be considered in all women of childbearing age complaining of abdominal pain. In the recent Confidential Enquiry into Maternal Deaths, ectopic pregnancy was listed as the fourth leading cause of direct deaths in pregnancy. Incidence of ectopic pregnancy in the UK is 11.1 per 1000 estimated pregnancies.

Presentation may be with any or all of the following: abdominal pain, shoulder tip pain due to diaphragmatic irritation, faintness or collapse. A pelvic mass may be palpable. Transvaginal ultrasound may reveal the same mass, or, more commonly, free fluid in the pouch of Douglas in the presence of an empty uterus.

If there is any clinical suspicion of an ectopic pregnancy, beta-hCG (human chorionic gonadotrophin) levels should be measured in maternal serum on two occasions 48 h apart. During the first 6–7 weeks of pregnancy, the level will double every 48 h in 90 per cent of pregnancies. (*Why Mothers Die*, 2001; *Obstetric and Gynecologic Secrets*, 1997)

267.

A. **True.** It suppresses the midcycle surge of gonadotrophins, and because of its long half-life it can be administered twice per week.
B. **False.** Gestrinone, like danazol and other progestogens, tends to decrease libido.
C. **True.** Voice changes and cliteromegaly are often irreversible, unlike most of its many other side effects.
D. **False.**

268.

A. **True.**

B. **False.** It reduces the incidence.

C. **False.**

D. **True.** And promotes peripheral blood flow by decreasing vascular resistance.

E. **False.** Lowers total and low-density lipoprotein and raises high-density lipoprotein, which may contribute to the reported reduction of approximately 50 per cent in the risk of coronary heart disease in HRT users.

F. **False.** 2 mg of oral oestradiol; 0.625 mg of conjugated equine oestrogens and 50 mg transdermally.

G. **True.** In older age, the use of oestrogen still produces a reduction in bone loss. After 10 years it is wise to assess the anticipated benefits of continuing HRT against the increased risk of breast cancer.

H. **False.** Tibolone has combined oestrogenic, progestogenic and androgenic effects and provides an alternative for women who require HRT but wish to avoid withdrawal bleeds. FSH levels are significantly suppressed and tibolone provides effective relief from vasomotor symptoms.

HRT benefits

Patients who exhibit one or more of the following risk factors should be considered for oestrogen replacement therapy:

- Low body weight.
- Increased blood pressure.
- Cigarette smoking.
- Alcohol.
- Hyperlipidaemia.
- Strong family history of cardiovascular disease.
- Low-impact fracture.
- Established osteoporosis.

269.

A. **True.** PAPS includes patients with lupus anticoagulant and ACA who are at increased risk of first and second trimester loss.

B. **False.** They are at increased risk of venous and arterial thromboembolism.

270.

A. **True.**

B. **False.**

C. **False.**

D. **True.**

E. **True.**

Female sexual dysfunction

There are various classifications of female sexual dysfunction. The main causes are vaginismus, lack of libido (which may be primary or secondary), difficulty in reaching orgasm (which may be primary or secondary), vaginal dryness or soreness – often linked to infection or loss of oestrogen pre or post-menopause. Sildenafil has not been very successful in women.

Simple counselling and psychotherapy are very helpful and will sort out most couples. Masters and Johnson pioneered the technique in USA. In the UK, the Institute of Psychosexual Medicine is influenced by Dr. Michael Balint and uses simple psychotherapy.

Reference: What's happening in female sexual dysfunction? *Trends in Urology, Gynaecology and Sexual Health* 2001; **6**: 12–13.

271.

A. **False.** Rupture of the fetal membranes (ROM) before the onset of labour is termed premature rupture of membranes (PROM), whether or not this rupture occurred before term, at term, or post-term. When it occurs before term it is termed preterm PROM. This occurs in 4–18 per cent of pregnancies and is responsible for nearly 50 per cent of the preterm deliveries, and consequently for 10 per cent of perinatal mortalities. Another consequence of PROM is an increase in infant morbidity and obstetric interventions. Complications can be severe, such as amnionitis, endometritis and puerperal sepsis in the mother, and neonatal sepsis in the newborn.

B. **False.** Frequently. The incidence of subclinical chorioamnionitis may be as high as 30 per cent. ROM is occasionally the result of an aggressive external factor (e.g. amniocentesis), but is usually due to the lack of resistance of the fetal membranes to the intra-amniotic pressure. No single factor has been identified.

C. **False.** Increases prostaglandins. There is increasing evidence of the major role of infection in PROM. On the one hand, it could produce a decrease in the resistance of connective tissue by means of direct protease and phospholipase bacterial production. On the other hand, it could increase production of prostaglandins, with an increase in uterine activity. Various studies of intra-amniotic infection have shown 20–40 per cent of positive cultures in preterm PROM.

D. **False.** Unless there is evidence of amniotic fluid in the vagina (pressing on the uterine fundus, or the Valsalva manoeuvre may help) there is often doubt. Confirmation must be obtained before aggressive action can be taken.

E. **False.** In cases of PROM at 36 or more weeks of gestation, the best solution is delivery. It will occur spontaneously in more than 80 per cent of cases within the first 24 h. If the cervix is favourable, induction of labour after 24–48 h is recommended in most centres.

F. **True.** And the difficulty in obtaining cultures in the newborn is overcome.

G. **True.** Lactobacilli being numerically dominant, while anaerobic bacteria are reduced.

272.

A. **True.** Other tocolytics include ritodrine, terbutaline, indomethacin, nifedipine and atosiban.

B. **False.** The efficacy of oral tocolytics is questionable, unlike the intravenous preparations.

C. **True.** It is thought that beta-agonists increase the amount of cyclic AMP in the muscle cells, reducing intracellular calcium and rendering the myosin–actin unit less sensitive to calcium.

D. **False.** The oral and intravenous fluid volume is restricted when tocolytics are used because of the risk of pulmonary oedema.

E. **True.** Insulin requirements are increased. Both steroids and beta-agonists are diabetogenic.

273.

A. **True.**

B. **True.** Preterm births are the major cause of perinatal mortality and morbidity in the developed world, and account for 8–10 per cent of all births.

C. **True.** And prolonged rupture and very little amniotic fluid.

D. **True.** Treatment with antenatal steroids reduces the risk of respiratory distress syndrome, intraventricular haemorrhage and necrotizing enterocolitis.

E. **False.** Preterm delivery accounts for 85 per cent once congenital abnormality is excluded.

F. **True.** Preterm delivery and subsequent physiological instability can lead to bleeding from the subependymal germinal matrix causing a periventricular haemorrhage (PVH). In its mildest form, the bleeding is limited to the germinal matrix-subependymal haemorrhage; with a moderate bleed, it extends into the lateral ventricles, and intraventricular haemorrhage, when the ventricles may also become dilated.

G. **True.** Ischaemic brain injury is often associated with periventricular haemorrhage. This cerebral hypoxic injury can be secondary to low arterial oxygen tension, hypotension, or reduced cerebral blood flow. All of these can be directly related to the infant's prematurity, or they can be iatrogenic. Long-term neurological sequelae are common.

H. **True.** 33 per cent at 23 weeks and 16 per cent at 24 weeks.

274.

A. **False.** The ratio is less than 0.5 at 20 weeks. A value of 2 indicates a low risk of respiratory distress syndrome at any point in gestation.

B. **False.** Lecithin and other phosphatidyl-lipids are produced by type II pneumocytes.

C. **False.** The L/S ratio is not reliable in the presence of blood or meconium.

D. **False.** This occurs between 23 and 24 weeks.

E. **True.** And type II pneumocytes are concerned with surfactant production.

F. **True.** BPD is caused by aberrant development in the immature lung secondary to positive-pressure ventilation and high-inspired oxygen concentration.

G. **False.** 95 per cent of babies born below 25 weeks develop CLD, and 5 per cent at 30 weeks.

275.

A. **False.** It is characterized by painless cervical dilatation.
B. **True.** In-utero exposure to diethlystilbestrol carries a 45 per cent risk of pregnancy loss. Diethylstilboestrol is a non-steroidal synthetic oestrogen. Increased frequencies of preterm labour, miscarriages and ectopic pregnancy have been reported among women whose mothers used DES during pregnancy (daughters of DES).
C. **False.** It is rarely associated.
D. **False.** Ritodrine alone will not stop the contractions.

276.

A. **False.** Problems encountered by preterm infants include thermal stress due to their high surface area-to-mass ratio. Thin skin allows high transudative water loss and heat loss by evaporation.
B. **False.** Surfactant production decreases as the infant's temperature drops.
C. **False.** Temperature drops cause an increase in oxygen and glucose consumption. Chances of survival can be increased by about 20 per cent when nursed in warmer thermoneutral environments.

277.

A. **True.**
B. **False.** 15 per cent of cases.
C. **True.**
D. **False.** Such tumours are usually well differentiated, with minimal invasiveness.
E. **True.** These patients are at increased risk of recurrence and death.

278.

A. **True.** Other benign conditions may lead to raised levels of Ca125: these include PID, endometriosis, pregnancy, TB, pericarditis and liver cirrhosis.
B. **True.** Ca125 is elevated in 50 per cent of stage I and 90 per cent of advanced ovarian cancer.
C. **True.**
D. **False.**
E. **True.** Ca125 may be raised with other tumours such as breast, lung, and colorectal.

279.

A. **False.** The miscarriage rate after amniocentesis is approximately 0.5–1.0 per cent, and it is greater before 15 weeks' gestation.
B. **True.** FISH takes 72 h to complete, while full karyotype results take 3 weeks.
C. **False.** The failure rate is 0.5–1.0 per cent. A further 0.25–1.0 per cent will show mosaicism, which is confirmed in only 50 per cent of fetuses.

280.

A. **True.** In addition, there is an increased incidence of renal and gastro-intestinal anomalies and severe mental retardation. The head may be small and elongated.
B. **True.**
C. **False.** Overlapping fingers. Polydactyly is a feature of trisomy 13, Patau's syndrome.
D. **True.**

> ## Trisomy
>
> ### Trisomy 18: Edward's syndrome:
>
> Incidence: 0.3 per 1000 newborns – increases with increasing maternal age.
>
> Features include small size, initial hypotonia, prominent occiput, small mouth, micrognathia, overlapping fingers, umbilical hernia, small pelvis, rockerbottom feet and cardiac defects.
>
> ### Trisomy 13: Patau's syndrome:
>
> Incidence: 1 per 5000 newborns – increases with increasing maternal age.
>
> Features include holoprosencephaly, deafness, microphthalmia, retinal dysplasia, cleft lip and palate, abnormal ears, polydactyly, hypoplasia of pelvis, exomphalos and cardiac defects.

281.

A. **True.** It occurs in 1:2500 live births.

B. **True.** 'Café au lait' patches are found on the skin, and neurofibromas develop on peripheral nerve sheaths.

C. **False.** 6 per cent is the risk of underlying malignancy

282.

A. **True.** General answer for A–D. Pre-implantation diagnosis (PGD) involves testing the early embryo after in-vitro fertilization. One or two blastomeres are removed at biopsy from the pre-implantation embryo at the 6- to 10-cell stage. Unaffected embryos are returned. It can be used for three major categories of disease: (1) sex-linked disorders, such as Duchenne's; (2) single gene defects, such as cystic fibrosis, where the molecular abnormality is testable with molecular techniques after polymerase chain reaction (PCR) amplification of DNA extracted from single cells; and (3) chromosomal disorders, where FISH (fluorescence in-situ hybridization) has been developed to detect a variety of chromosomal problems such as translocations, inversions and deletions.

B. **False.**

C. **True.**

D. **True.**

E. **False.** Approximately 15 per cent of newborns are thus affected. The incidence increases in multiple pregnancy.

283.

A. True.

B. False. In the majority of cases the cause is unknown. It is a self-extending process with the accumulating blood clot causing more separation. Blood can reach the amniotic cavity (by disrupting the placenta, producing blood-stained liquor) and the myometrium (Couvelaire uterus).

C. False. The cause of placental abruption is frequently unknown. In a few cases, however, it is obvious, such as in direct trauma to the uterus.

D. True. Despite, in many cases, considerable blood loss. It is uncertain whether the hypertension is a cause or a consequence of the abruption.

E. True. Because labour is the most common factor precipitating placental separation, nearly 50 per cent of patients are in established labour. The patient typically develops pain over the uterus, and this increases in severity. There is usually no periodicity until uterine contractions start and superimpose additional intermittent pain. Faintness and collapse may occur, as may signs of shock.

F. False.

284.

A. True.

B. True.

C. False. Liver enzymes are usually moderately elevated.

Acute fatty liver

The hepatic lesion is characterized by deposition of fat microdroplets within the hepatocytes. Inflammation and necrosis are usually absent, and some cases may be misdiagnosed as hepatitis.

285.

A. False. Great care must be taken when prescribing in women with acute porphyria. Progestogens are probably more hazardous than oestrogens.

B. False. Migraine sufferers can use oral progesterone-only contraception.

C. True. But it is safe to use in patients with peptic ulcer disease, bottle-feeding and endometriosis. In addition, it is contraindicated in patients with a history of undiagnosed vaginal bleeding and liver adenoma.

Porphyria

There are several different types of porphyria (acute intermittent porphyria, variegate porphyria, hereditary coproporphyria and 5-aminolaevulinic acid dehydratase deficiency porphyria). They are all a result of abnormalities in the metabolism of porphyrins, which are involved in the biosynthesis of haem. They have the prevalence of about 1 in 10 000 of the population.

Drugs unsafe for use in acute porphyrias:

Amphetamines, anabolic steroids, antidepressants, antihistamines, barbiturates, benzodiazepines, cephalosporins, contraceptive steroids, diuretics, ergot derivatives, gold salts, hormone replacement therapy, menopausal steroids, progestogens, sulphonamides and sulphonylureas.

References

British National Formulary (2001). British Medical Association, London.

CLASP collaborative group (1995). Low dose aspirin in pregnancy and early childhood development: follow up of the collaborative low dose aspirin study in pregnancy. *Br. J. Obstet. Gynaecol.*, **102**(11), 861–8.

DoH (1993). Report of the National Confidential Enquiry into Perioperative Deaths 1991/1992. HMSO, London.

Dewhurst's Textbook of Obstetrics and Gynaecology for Postgraduates (1995). 6th edition. Blackwell Scientific Publications, Oxford.

Frederickson, H.L. (1997). *Obstetric and Gynecologic Secrets*. Hanley & Belfus, USA.

ISSUD (1986). Report of the ISSUD Terminology Committee. *J. Reprod. Med.*, **31**: 973–4.

Jones, K. (1988). *Smith's Recognisable Patterns of Human Malformation*. 4th edition. W. B. Saunders Co., Philadelphia.

MAGPIE trial (2002). Do women with pre-eclampsia, and their babies, benefit from magnesium sulphate? The MAGPIE Trial: a randomized placebo-controlled trial. *Lancet*, **359**(9321): 1877–90.

Nagar, H. and Price, J. (2001). Screening in Epithelial Ovarian Cancer. *Northern Ireland Medicine Today*, June 2001.

Nyberg, D. (1990). *Diagnostic Ultrasound of Fetal Anomalies*. Mosby Year-Book, St Louis.

Polson, D.W., Franks, S., Reed, M.J., Cheng, R.W., Adams, J., James, V.H. (1987). The distribution of oestradiol in plasma in relation to uterine cross-sectional area in women with polycystic or multifollicular ovaries. *Clin. Endocrinol. (Oxf)*, **26**(5), 581–8.

RCOG Guidelines. Royal College of Obstetricians and Gynaecologists, London.

The British Journal of Obstetrics and Gynaecology (BJOG).

The Cochrane Library (www.cochrane.org).

The Progress Series: Progress in Obstetrics and Gynaecology (Studd, J., ed.).

Vacca, A. (1992). *Handbook of Vacuum Extraction in Obstetric Practice*. Edward Arnold, London.

WHO (1997). Intrauterine devices: technical and managerial guidelines for services.

Why Mothers Die (2001). Report on Confidential Enquiries into Maternal Deaths in the United Kingdom. HMSO, London.

Index

A denotes information in the Answers section